Breaking the Bonds
—— of ——
Irritable Bowel Syndrome

A psychological approach to
regaining control of your life

Barbara Bradley Bolen, Ph.D.

Foreword by W. Grant Thompson, M.D.
Emeritus Professor of Medicine, University of Ottawa

Copyright © 2010 Barbara Bradley Bolen
All rights reserved.
ISBN: 145633199X
ISBN-13: 9781456331993

For my boys.

Contents

	Foreword	7
	Acknowledgments	9
	Introduction	11
1	Understanding Your Digestive System	17
2	Feeling Good about Your Medical Care	29
3	Food is Not the Enemy!	45
4	Taking Aim at Acute Symptoms	65
5	Dealing with Difficult Situations	79
6	Improving Your Emotional Awareness	95
7	Monitoring Your Thoughts	113
8	A Calm Mind in a Calm Body	127
9	The Proactive Approach: Building Skills and Breaking Free	143
10	Beyond IBS: Developing a Healthy Lifestyle	161
	Resources	173
	References	175

Foreword

You might be wondering whether this book will be able to help you with the distressing intestinal symptoms of irritable bowel syndrome (IBS). Rest assured: Dr. Barbara Bradley Bolen has designed a program to help people whose lives are compromised by the symptoms and the need to cope with them. IBS isn't like peptic ulcers, cancer, or heart disease—it doesn't damage organs, threaten life, or prompt a surgical or pharmacological countermeasure. It is a disease of symptoms, so we only know of the existence of the condition by what patients report. That's why words, thoughts, and feelings are paramount. It is in this area that Dr. Bolen's psychological approach can offer both comfort and practical assistance.

Irritable bowel syndrome consists of recurrent episodes of abdominal pain related to altered bowel habit, which may consist of predominantly constipation or diarrhea, or an alternation between the two. Bloating often prompts loosening of clothing, and sufferers may feel a lack of satisfaction after defecation and notice mucus in the stools. Because there is no structural abnormality in the gastrointestinal tract that can explain IBS, it is often referred to as a "functional" illness. We don't know the cause of IBS, but it is widely believed that the intestines are hypersensitive and overreact to stimuli that wouldn't be noticed by people without IBS.

IBS is found in about 15 percent of the population worldwide, and is the most common digestive complaint in primary care and gastroenterology clinics. Nevertheless, most people who have these complaints don't report them to doctors. Women are twice as likely to have these symptoms as men and four times as likely to report them to a doctor. Does this mean that IBS is more severe in women? Not necessarily! In India and Japan, men are several times more likely than women to consult a doctor for IBS.

Those who consult a physician may be worried about the meaning of the condition. Many are satisfied to know that they don't have cancer or another serious disease. The family doctor may give advice regarding diet and lifestyle and provide psychological support where necessary. Currently available drugs are of little help, but an antidiarrheal drug may help control episodes of diarrhea, and bran or a bulking material such as psyllium may help constipation.

Most patients seeing family doctors are satisfied with such treatment. Some who are unsatisfied are referred to specialists, usually gastroenterologists. Among those referred patients are those who have psychosocial difficulties, including depression, anxiety, and panic. It is especially these patients who need to "break the bonds of IBS." Once the gastroenterologist (or any doctor) is satisfied that the diagnosis is correct, that the diet is satisfactory, and that there is no coexisting medical disease, he or she must consider the need for a psychological approach. Dr. Bolen, a practicing psychologist, offers just such an approach in this book.

Dr. Bolen's outgoing and conversational writing style make *Breaking the Bonds of IBS* easy to read and understand. Her positive approach (using IBS as a prompt for better emotional health), gentle humor, and practical steps make this a valuable manual for the troubled IBS patient. Gastroenterologists have much to learn from Dr. Bolen's writing as well, and will want to recommend it to their patients. I wish I had had her assistance with the many people I have seen over thirty-one years of practice whose working and private lives were disrupted by IBS. Her book is the next best thing.

—W. Grant Thompson, M.D.
Emeritus Professor of Medicine,
University of Ottawa

Acknowledgments

A special acknowledgment for the help of all the lovely California voices of New Harbinger who helped me with the process of having this book published. Thanks to Kristin Beck, Acquisitions Manager, and Jueli Gastwirth, Acquisitions Editor, for their enthusiastic encouragement and support. Much gratitude is extended to Heather Garnos, Senior Editor, whose breadth of knowledge, attention to detail, and jazzy headings helped to make this book the best that it could be.

An additional note of thanks to Dr. Grant Thompson for going above and beyond the call of duty in writing the foreword. His kind words and editorial suggestions are much appreciated.

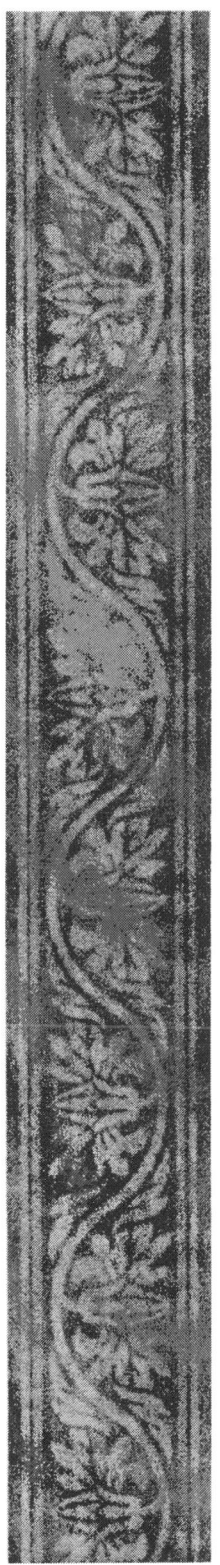

INTRODUCTION

A pretty young woman sat in my office, crying. She told me that she had been asked to be a bridesmaid at a wedding that was to take place at the Plaza Hotel in New York City. Instead of feeling honored, she was terrified. Instead of envisioning the excitement of such an experience, all she could think about was being trapped in a limousine, petrified that she might have an accident. Instead of anticipating the glamour of participating in a ceremony held at one of the world's most beautiful hotels, she could only picture being unable to get access to a bathroom, with all eyes upon her. Listening to her, I was once again struck by how debilitating irritable bowel syndrome can be. With that thought, however, comes the comfort of knowing how *treatable* IBS is.

What Is IBS?

So, you too are suffering from the woes of irritable bowel syndrome. You know all too well what the symptoms are: abdominal pain only relieved by having a bowel movement, chronic swings between diarrhea and constipation, feeling bloated and miserable. You are overwhelmed by how these symptoms have taken over your life. You are disgusted by having to deal so directly with these bodily functions that you would much rather ignore. You are terrified that maybe there's something more seriously wrong with you, and you wonder if perhaps the doctors have missed something.

For what it's worth, you aren't alone. It is estimated that irritable bowel syndrome affects anywhere from 10 to 20 percent of the population. Although it's not life-threatening, IBS is not an insignificant health problem. IBS sufferers account for a majority of visits to gastroenterologists, and the syndrome is a major reason for days missed from work.

Despite the prevalence of IBS, most people feel fairly alone in their suffering. Unfortunately, our society is still not comfortable talking openly about our intestines. Although IBS is common, people rarely divulge that they are struggling with the disorder. At most, you might hear someone say that they have "tummy trouble." The effort to cover up symptoms and the corresponding feelings of shame and embarrassment can serve to further exacerbate those very same symptoms and the discomfort that goes along with them.

What is this beast that has taken over your life? Irritable bowel syndrome is called a "functional" disorder of the intestinal system, meaning that there's something wrong with the way the system is functioning, as opposed to any visible disease process or tissue damage. The nasty symptoms that you're experiencing appear to be related to two factors. The first has to do with the speed of the motor functioning of your gut, with the system moving too quickly (resulting in diarrhea), or too slowly (causing constipation). The other factor is an increased sensitivity to a variety of triggers, which may cause hyperreactivity to pain, hormones, certain foods, and stressful situations.

Your next question is likely to be, "Why did this happen to me?" Although we don't currently know why some people develop IBS and others are spared, researchers have found some clues. One interesting finding is that some people experience a severe bout of what is commonly called the stomach flu, or gastroenteritis, prior to the onset of IBS. It is thought that the severe diarrhea caused by the gastroenteritis results in the intestinal hyperreactivity seen in irritable bowel syndrome. It has also been found that many IBS patients have experienced a significantly stressful event shortly before becoming symptomatic. It may be that the toll that this type of experience takes on the body manifests itself in a bowel dysfunction. One last clue has to do with the fact that a large number of IBS patients have a coexisting emotional illness, such as an anxiety disorder or depression. Although the painful and intrusive nature of IBS symptoms would certainly cause almost anyone to feel anxious and depressed, it is also thought that a central nervous system dysfunction (such as an imbalance of certain brain chemicals) may contribute to both the mood and the intestinal symptoms.

The good news about irritable bowel syndrome is that it is generally associated with a good prognosis. There is no evidence that IBS leads to any more serious diseases, nor does it decrease your life expectancy. There is no need for surgery, and IBS does not increase your risk for cancer. IBS is also quite treatable. Study after study shows that, with treatment, IBS symptoms abate, and that this symptom reduction continues to manifest itself after treatment has ended.

Mind Over Matter

The most unhelpful words ever spoken are "It's all in your head." On good days, you yourself may think, "Maybe I'm imagining that it's really as bad as it is." Then you find yourself doubled over on the toilet bowl and you know that you aren't making this up. So, you may be wondering, if this isn't all in your head, how can a psychologist help?

First of all, you have become the unfortunate victim of a chronic illness. Life is hard enough without having to deal with an unpredictable body. It is easy to begin to feel overwhelmed, as if you are falling apart. You may also be feeling some of the isolation that we talked about earlier. Psychologists are experts at helping people to deal with this kind of stress.

Although IBS shares many of the same characteristics that make any chronic illness difficult to deal with, my experience has been that IBS comes with its own set of specific psychological aftereffects. By this I mean certain distressing negative emotions that are triggered by the painful and unpleasant symptoms of IBS. To illustrate this, let me tell you about a patient of mine. Mary Lou is a thirty-two-year-old travel agent. Although her work involves helping others to plan their dream vacation, Mary Lou has been grounded by IBS. Due to a fear of having pain and diarrhea while out in public, Mary Lou has developed an agoraphobic-like avoidance and will only travel short distances from her home. Even then, she must be the one doing the driving so that she knows she can quickly drive herself home should she need to use the bathroom. Her anticipatory anxiety, i.e., worrying ahead of time about what might happen, is so severe that she is unable to commit to any type of planned or scheduled social event. Thus, her IBS has resulted in significant psychological distress for which psychological treatment is clearly indicated.

A psychological approach is also essential if you are one of those IBS sufferers who is coping with a coexisting mood disorder. Psychological treatment has repeatedly been shown to be quite effective for depression and a variety of anxiety disorders. Similarly, if you are one of those people whose IBS manifested itself following a significant psychosocial stressor, you will find that a psychologist's expertise in stress management and helping people to work through losses goes a long way toward helping you to feel better both physically and emotionally.

An Active Approach

In my practice I utilize what is called a cognitive behavioral approach to treatment. Cognitive behavioral treatment has been shown to be quite effective for a wide variety of disorders, including irritable bowel syndrome. Cognitive behavioral treatment involves teaching people healthier ways of thinking and healthier ways of behaving in order to help people to *feel* better. This approach has alway appealed to me because it is very active and practical, with a focus on teaching skills to improve a person's ability to manage their life successfully. Attention is given to present-day problems, looking to the past only as it is affecting one's current functioning. With this approach, I see my role as that of a coach. You are the one who is out there living your life, and currently coping with a painful illness, but I can teach you strategies to help you to manage your IBS and your life more effectively. The larger goals of treatment are greater life satisfaction and improved quality of life.

Charting a Course to Recovery

Within the cognitive behavioral framework, I have found one of the most helpful tools to be the use of simple charts for monitoring the relationship between unpleasant symptoms and external triggers. Triggers can consist of foods eaten, stressful events, certain emotional states, and even unhealthy ways of thinking. Keeping track of these triggers helps you to figure out what sorts of things help you to feel better and what sorts of things make you feel worse. This information goes a long way toward helping you to regain some sense of control. And control is a wonderful thing, and with a chronic and unpredictable illness like IBS it at times feels like a rare commodity. Self-monitoring is a wonderful device for bringing back the feeling that you're in charge of your own life.

Throughout this book, I will be presenting you with forms to fill out to help you to track your symptoms, improve your emotional awareness, and identify and challenge unhealthy thoughts. Each of these factors will be recorded in turn and eventually you will be using a self-monitoring sheet that includes a column entitled Coping Skills. My job is to teach you the strategies that you will need to confidently fill in this column. You will learn how to successfully assert yourself, how to use relaxation techniques to reduce anxiety and muscle tension, and how to prioritize and delegate your responsibilities so as to manage your stress better. You will experience a tremendous sense of accomplishment as you utilize new skills and capitalize on your existing strengths to break free of the restrictions placed upon you by this oh-so-disruptive digestive disorder.

The Silver Lining

From all bad things comes some good, and IBS is no exception. Although you will certainly never be grateful that IBS has come into your life, the long-term effect of this experience can be a positive one. The benefits of reading this book, completing the exercises, and developing new skills go way beyond coping with irritable bowel syndrome. Your improved emotional awareness, ability to think more clearly, and newfound skills for relaxing or asserting yourself will have a significant positive effect on your overall mental health.

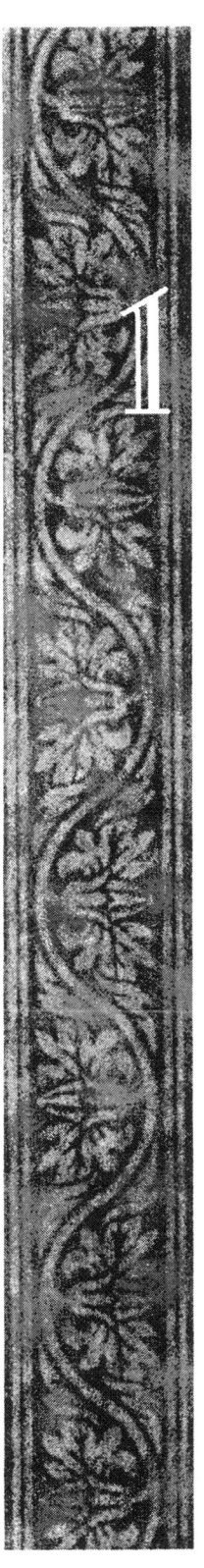

1 Understanding Your Digestive System

Remember those long, hot afternoons when you were stuck sitting in high school biology? If you were anything like me, you'd sit there wondering, "When in my life am I ever going to need to know this stuff?" Well, high school is coming back to haunt you. Believe it or not, becoming reacquainted with what you learned when you were fifteen years old is actually going to help you feel better.

Information Is Power

Think about how you feel when your car starts acting up. If you know a lot about cars, you know that you could fix it yourself or feel fairly confident that you are getting a straight story from your mechanic. If you know relatively little about cars, you might feel vulnerable and powerless when you have to take yours to the shop. Having knowledge about how something works affects your ability to deal with it when it doesn't. Your body is certainly experiencing some engine trouble, and learning about what is happening is the first step toward regaining control over your life.

It is vital that you understand how your digestive system is supposed to work—and why yours isn't working that way. This information will help you in many ways. Visualizing the process that leads to your symptoms helps you to remember that symptom flare-ups do come to an end! When you are experiencing acute symptoms, knowing what your gastrointestinal tract is doing can help you to visualize the malfunction working its way through your system until it eventually comes to a stop. Listen to what Edward, a thirty-year-old computer programmer, had to say about this. Edward had only recently been diagnosed with irritable bowel syndrome when he came to my office for his initial psychotherapy appointment. He said, "The first thing I did after getting diagnosed was to go to the library and take out a book on the digestive system. Although I still felt miserable, it really helped me to picture what was going on inside me. By imagining the process that was causing all that painful cramping I was able to keep reminding myself that the symptoms would eventually die down and I would feel better."

Information also helps to get rid of the unknowns, those scary things that we all spend so much time worrying about. Knowing that you don't have cancer will keep you somewhat calmer even when you absolutely feel like you are dying. Because symptom flare-ups of IBS can be so debilitating and distressing, it is quite common to fear that something more serious, e.g. life threatening, has been overlooked. Having an understanding of how a diagnosis of irritable bowel syndrome is reached will help you to have confidence that you have not been misdiagnosed.

Information will help to motivate you to make the healthy lifestyle choices that you need to make in order to better manage your IBS. Understanding how the food that you eat, the thoughts that you think, and the way you cope with the stresses in your life affect your intestinal system will help you to actively work to make changes in these areas.

Last, but not least, possessing basic information about your body and your IBS will help you to work more comfortably with your doctor. Just like with a mechanic, understanding the framework that the expert is working in helps to instill trust. Having a good working relationship with your doctor is an essential factor in your efforts to work toward wellness. Possessing basic information about your gastrointestinal system and irritable bowel syndrome will help you to ask informed questions, speak confidently about your concerns, and express doubts if something your doctor has said doesn't sit well with you.

This knowledge served one of my patients quite well. Karen had gone to see her internist after she first began to experience episodes of painful cramping and diarrhea. Her doctor prescribed a variety of diagnostic tests, including a colonoscopy. Karen was reluctant to schedule the colonoscopy due to her history of difficulty tolerating sedation. Karen was a nurse, and she decided to ask one of the doctors on staff in the hospital where she worked what he thought. He told her that because she was only twenty-seven and not in any risk group for colon cancer, he thought the test was unnecessary and that a diagnosis of irritable bowel syndrome could be made with confidence without the colonoscopy. He recommended that Karen see a gastroenterologist for a second opinion. Karen took his advice, and her gastroenterologist assured her that a colonoscopy was not needed. Karen was greatly relieved. Her story clearly illustrates the advantage of being an educated patient. A knowledge of basic biology will reduce your sense of vulnerability, soothe some of your anxiety, and begin to help you to feel better.

Flashback to High School!

Let's see how good your memory is as we review the digestive system. Prepare yourself. Talking about the digestive system automatically involves using words like rectum, stool, and diarrhea. There is just no way around it. Unfortunately, our civilized society has branded these words taboo in polite conversation, and so being exposed to them sometimes elicits uncomfortable feelings. Hopefully, you are not too squeamish.

Nuts and Bolts

You can picture the digestive system, a.k.a. the gastrointestinal system, as being like a long conveyor belt that extends from your mouth all the way through to your rectum. See what I mean? Just using mouth and rectum in the same sentence may be enough to make you squirm. Anyway, digestion begins in your mouth as you chew your food. Saliva, which moistens the food, also contains enzymes that begin the process of breaking down starches and fats. The act of swallowing pushes the food into the esophagus which, in turn, moves the food down into your stomach.

Your stomach's job is to store, break up, and churn your meal. The stomach releases pepsin, an enzyme that helps with the digestion of protein, and hydrochloric acid, which kills bacteria and breaks the food up into a substance called chyme. Approximately two to three hours after food is eaten, the chyme is slowly released into the small intestine.

The small intestine is responsible for the absorption of all essential nutrients into the bloodstream. It is thought that some of the motor speed difficulties seen in IBS start right here in the small intestine. In its work, the small intestine is aided by those other organs, the ones you always hear about but may have no idea what they do, namely the liver, gallbladder, and pancreas. The liver produces bile and stores it in the gallbladder, which releases the bile into the small intestine as needed. In the small intestine, bile surrounds fat cells and dissolves them into a liquid that can be absorbed by the body. The pancreas releases enzymes that are highly alkaline and thus serve to neutralize the hydrochloric acid from the stomach. These same enzymes also work to break down proteins, carbohydrates, and fats.

Hang in there! We're almost through. The small intestine is made up of three parts: the duodenum, the jejunum, and the ileum. Bile from the gallbladder and secretions from the pancreas are added to the chyme in the duodenum. Fats, starches, and proteins are broken down and absorbed in the jejunum. Calcium, minerals, and vitamins are absorbed in the ileum. The small intestine is really quite a powerhouse!

Any leftover material is passed into the large intestine otherwise known as the colon. The colon's main job is to extract water and salt from this leftover material and compact it so that it can be eliminated. The material moves through the cecum, the ascending colon, the transverse colon, and then the descending colon. Once or twice a day the stool is moved into the lowest part of the colon, the sigmoid colon. The stool's presence in the sigmoid colon puts pressure on the rectum and results in the urge to move your bowels.

The Mind-Body Link

It is also important to know a little bit about the relationship between your brain and your digestive system. The gut seems to have its own brain, called the enteric nervous system, which governs the process of digestion. The enteric nervous system (ENS) is comprised of nerves within the walls of the intestines with connections to the muscles and blood vessels. The hormones and neurotransmitters within the ENS affect the workings of the whole system. The ENS is directly connected to the brain through nerves that pass through the spinal cord to the base of the brain. This communication network is a two-way street: thus, messages are sent directly back and forth from the brain to the digestive system. It is in this manner that our intestines appear to become hypersensitive in response to outside stress.

The whole process sounds relatively uncomplicated, right? So why have your bowels gone haywire? Modern medicine doesn't yet have an answer as to what causes irritable bowel syndrome, but some contributing factors have been identified. Keep in mind that IBS is a functional disease, that is, there is something wrong with the way that the system works, as opposed to a structural disease, in which there is observable inflammation or tissue damage.

The Ills of IBS

Now, here's an area in which you are already an expert: namely, the symptoms of IBS. In order for IBS to be diagnosed, symptoms must be chronic and persistent, and must have been present for at least three months. The most common symptoms are abdominal pain and a change in the frequency and consistency of bowel movements. Abdominal pain is generally relieved by defecation. Bloating and a perception of excessive gas are common. Another symptom is the presence of mucus in the stool.

IBS tends to manifest itself in one of two ways, either diarrhea-predominant or constipation-predominant. If your IBS is constipation-predominant, you may find yourself straining when having a bowel movement. With diarrhea, there may be an urgent need to get to a bathroom.

With both conditions, there may be a sensation after defecation that you have not completely emptied your bowels.

Lovely stuff, huh? Sometimes people with IBS feel that other people, including doctors, do not take them seriously. It might be reassuring to know that medical researchers take IBS quite seriously and have been working hard to identify what is going wrong so they can figure out how to develop helpful treatment protocols. The following sections will cover some of the most recent and pertinent findings. You will see that there is ample evidence that this is *not* just all in your head.

So What's Going on in There?

Laboratory studies that compare the digestive systems of people who are diagnosed with IBS to people who have other digestive disorders—or to those lucky souls who are healthy—have found two significant differences. It has been found that people with IBS experience abnormal visceral sensitivity and motility dysfunction. Let me explain what that means.

Increased Sensation

Viscera are internal organs. Thus, abnormal visceral sensitivity refers to the fact that people with IBS have intestines that are especially sensitive and react with pain to the material that is passing through. If you think you have problems, listen to what research subjects have consented to: In order to mimic the sensation of gas or stool in the intestine, balloons were inserted at various parts of the system and then slowly filled with air. (Talk about sacrifice for the sake of science!) Measurements were taken regarding the amount of discomfort a person feels at various pressure levels. These balloon distension studies consistently indicated that IBS patients experience intestinal pain at a lower pressure level than nonpatients (Mayer and Gebhart 1994).

Now, scientists are no dummies. They thought "Maybe IBS patients are just oversensitive to pain in general." To test this, they compared the response of IBS patients and nonpatients to other forms of uncomfortable stimulation. This type of comparison shows that IBS patients actually have a *greater* tolerance for pain experienced at other parts of the body (Cook, van Eeden, and Collins 1987). Thus, it appears that there is some alteration in the intestines of IBS patients that results in the abdominal pain that is felt in response to the presence of gas or stool.

Motility Problems

Motility refers to the speed of the movement of the gastrointestinal muscles. Research has consistently demonstrated motility difficulties in the intestines of IBS patients (Thompson 1993). When diarrhea is active, motility is characterized by a higher number of fast contractions, resulting in a rapid transit time for stool material. Constipation is characterized by intestinal contractions that are fewer and slower. These motility difficulties appear to start in the small intestine and continue on through the entire system.

An interesting study was conducted by a group of researchers (Kellow, Gill, and Wingate 1990) who studied the intestinal motility of subjects for three days. They found that the clustered intestinal contractions that differentiate IBS patients from nonpatients were only seen when the subjects were awake. This explains why IBS flare-ups rarely wake a person from sleep. More importantly, it points to the role that the perception of outside stress plays in triggering IBS symptoms.

A Higher Connection

As IBS manifests itself in dysfunction of both visceral sensitivity and motility, it is thought that perhaps there is some common problem that contributes to both. Scientists are thus looking at the central nervous system (brain) as a potential culprit. A central nervous system dysfunction would explain the frequent coexistence of IBS and psychiatric diagnoses. Further compelling evidence for a central problem comes from the fact that many IBS sufferers also have correlated difficulties with other parts of the body, namely the esophagus, stomach, bladder, and vagina (Farthing 1995). What these organs have in common is that they are all comprised of smooth muscle. Thus there may be an underlying condition that contributes to the symptoms experienced throughout the body.

This correlation came as a great relief to one of my patients. Elaine is a forty-five-year-old working mother of three, who in addition to coping with IBS, was constantly struggling with urinary tract pain. "I was really beginning to doubt myself," she said. "Was I turning into a hypochondriac? I find that I'm constantly in the bathroom, going one way or the other. It makes me feel a little better to think that I am perhaps just dealing with one problem and am not going crazy."

Stress Counts . . .

In addition to looking at the physiological differences of IBS patients, scientists have examined the relationship between various factors and the onset of IBS. The most obvious of these is stress. Creed, Craig, and Farmer (1988) looked at the relationship between significantly stressful life events and the onset of a functional gastrointestinal disorder such as IBS. The functional gastrointestinal disorder sufferers were significantly more likely to have experienced a major life stressor, such as the breakup of a relationship, prior to the onset of their condition than were a group of patients undergoing an appendectomy or a group of healthy patients. Another study (Whitehead et al. 1992) evaluated the stress levels of IBS patients compared to a group of individuals with some bowel difficulties and a group of nonsymptomatic people. This comparison took place over a year's time. They found that IBS patients experienced significantly higher stress levels over the course of the year than did the other two groups. Thus, IBS may be precipitated by an extremely stressful experience or exacerbated by ongoing life stressors.

Take a Look Back

Think about your own recent past. Have you experienced a major life event, such as a marital separation or divorce, a death, or a major job change? This event may have taken a grave toll on your body. Now think about your life. Are you dealing with more stress than is healthy? Do you think this is contributing to the way that you feel? For many people the answer to these questions is obvious. For others the focus on physical symptoms serves to mask life problems that may be too threatening to face.

Marty had no difficulty identifying the stress that contributed to his IBS. He was first plagued by the disorder when he left his corporate job to start up his own insurance agency. "Ask my wife. I was completely stressed out. I was so worried that I wasn't going to be able to support my family and pay the mortgage. That first year in business was so tough. My system did not handle the stress well. I went to the doctor every other week because I was so sick that I thought there had to be something more seriously wrong."

Roberta was a different story. She was a housewife with grown children. When she first came to see me, at the request of her gastroenterologist, all she could talk about was how bad her IBS had gotten. Although she had always had, in her words, a "sensitive system," lately she felt that she could no longer cope with it. She was convinced that something had changed with her physically even though all diagnostic procedures had turned up negative. It took a while, but Roberta eventually acknowledged how deeply she had been affected by her youngest child's recent marriage, which left Roberta with an empty nest after many years of attending to the needs of her children. Roberta also began to get in touch with how serious her husband's drinking had become and the effects that this was having on her. As she worked in therapy to come to grips with psychosocial stressors, her intestinal symptoms diminished.

But Stress Isn't the Only Thing

Researchers have also focused on the role that personality factors and psychological distress play in the development of IBS. You'll probably be glad to hear that IBS patients do not differ psychologically from people who suffer other identified, organic gastrointestinal illnesses (Smith et al. 1990). Differences *are* found between those who seek medical treatment and those who do not. People who cope with their IBS on their own don't differ psychologically from healthy individuals, but those who seek medical treatment for their IBS generally demonstrate significantly more psychological distress (Drossman et al. 1988).

A history of having been physically or sexually abused has been associated with a vulnerability toward the development of IBS. One study (Drossman et al. 1990) found that nearly half of the individuals seen at a gastroenterology practice reported a history of physical or sexual abuse. Patients with functional gastrointestinal disorders reported significantly more episodes of physical and sexual abuse than did those who were diagnosed with organic disorders. It is not yet known if IBS and abuse are connected. It is possible that exposure to repeated traumatic experiences results in a breakdown in the way that the body deals with stress. People who were abused in childhood are also more likely to experience psychiatric symptoms. Chronic physical difficulties and mood disorders appear to be some of the enduring scars from early trauma.

As discussed previously, another possible contributing factor to the development of IBS has to do with the experience of a bad case of what is commonly called the stomach flu. A recent study (Neal, Hebden, and Spiller 1997) surveyed a large group of people who had confirmed cases of infectious bacterial gastroenteritis and found that one-quarter of these individuals still experienced altered bowel functioning six months later. Approximately 10 percent of those studied went on to develop a diagnosed case of irritable bowel syndrome, with women being at particular risk. If you feel that you fall into this category, take heart. It is thought that IBS that is preceded by gastroenteritis is associated with a better prognosis and a quicker return to health.

Food intolerance is another contributing factor in the onset of irritable bowel syndrome. A food intolerance results when the intestines do not absorb certain substances found in food. When these substances enter the colon, they are attacked by bacteria, resulting in the production of gas, which contributes to abdominal pain and cramping. The unabsorbed material can contribute to diarrhea. It has been estimated that up to 40 percent of IBS patients experience lactose intolerance. Other food intolerances are fairly rare, but certain foods and food additives (such as caffeine and the artificial sweetener sorbitol) may trigger symptoms in some individuals.

Are Women at Higher Risk?

In America, women seek treatment for IBS two to three times as often as do men. One possible explanation has to do with the role that hormones play in exacerbating IBS symptoms. Although most women experience some gastrointestinal symptoms during menstruation, this change is seen more significantly in women with IBS (Whitehead et al. 1990). One more thing to blame on PMS!

Women are also more likely than men to suffer from depression. As IBS and depression often go hand in hand, a chemical imbalance contributing to both disorders may explain the greater number of women who seek treatment for IBS. Women are also more likely than men to have experienced sexual trauma. Again, it is possible that there is a common link. One last possible explanation has to do with the fact that women, in general, are less comfortable with the workings of their gastrointestinal system. Thus, they may experience more distress from bloating, gas, and time spent in the bathroom than men do. Think about your own childhood. If someone were to openly pass gas, wasn't that someone likely to be your father? Most women are mortified by such an experience. This socialized discomfort may make it more likely for women to see a doctor for diagnosis and treatment.

The Driver's Seat

Did you ever play the board game called Life? Do you remember those cute little cars with the pegs for people? Well, it is time to put your little peg back into the driver's seat of your life. You are now armed with solid information regarding the way your body works and some of the most up-to-date research as to why it is experiencing periodic breakdowns. Although you still have to cope with the unpredictability of symptom flare-ups, you have taken an important first step toward being in charge of the direction your life is taking.

Jeremy, a newly married accountant, said it best. "Thank you for telling me what is known so far about what causes IBS. Just because I'm not a doctor doesn't mean that I don't have a right to know what is going on with my body. The research findings make sense to me. They have really helped me to understand how my current stress level and my rocky childhood are most likely affecting how I am feeling. It's good to be on the road to recovery. It's nice to feel that I am now calling the shots again—not my doctor, and not my colon."

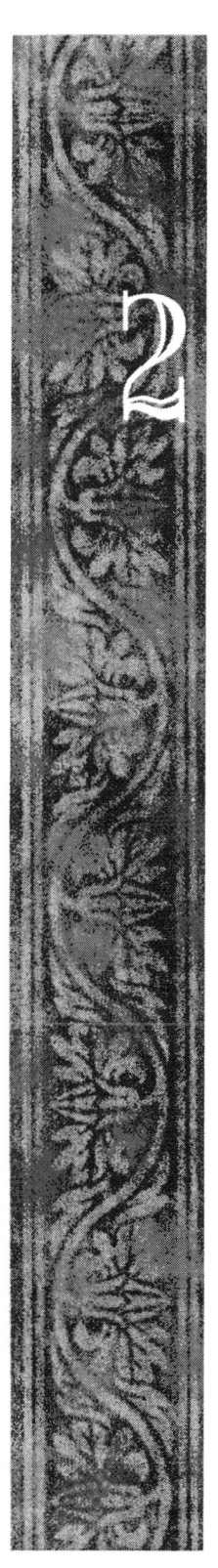

2 Feeling Good about Your Medical Care

Collaboration. I can't think of a word that more accurately describes the optimal relationship between a patient and their doctor. Collaboration involves working toward a common goal. In this case, the obvious goal is for you to feel better.

In sailboat racing, two of the most important jobs are those of the helmsperson and the tactician. The helmsperson is responsible for steering the boat toward victory. The tactician's job is to evaluate conditions and make recommendations regarding the best course of action. The helmsperson takes in this information but is ultimately responsible for making all decisions. This teamwork is essential for a successful outcome.

A healthy doctor-patient relationship works in much the same way. Your doctor, much like the tactican, is responsible for evaluating your symptoms and outlining treatment strategies. Your job is to use the feedback that you get from your doctor to steer a course to recovery. Like the helmsperson, you need to take in the information given to you and use it to your best advantage. Becoming acquainted with the framework that your doctor works in, the language that they use, and the information that they are looking for will strengthen your teamwork and maximize the outcome of your joint effort.

The Right Match

Hopefully you have already been seen and diagnosed by a qualified physician. If not, I urge you to do so at once. Accurate diagnosis is of the utmost importance, as other, more serious disorders share some of the same symptoms.

When it comes to your health, a good relationship with your doctor is important. When it comes to coping with IBS in particular, a good relationship with your doctor can make a significant difference in treatment outcome. When the people who invest big money in sailboat racing put together a crew, they spend a lot of time evaluating personalities and looking for team members who are a good fit. Since you'll be investing time and money into getting better, it is important that you make sure that you and your doctor are a good match. Therefore, be a good consumer! Find a doctor who seems knowledgeable and with whom you feel comfortable. Ann Landers recommends that people interview three therapists before beginning treatment. This advice is also applicable to choosing a gastroenterologist. Although few people are this thorough, her point is well taken. Don't just feel you have to be stuck with the first person that you consult. If you don't feel comfortable, try someone else until you find a person that you think you can work with.

Your first question might be, "What kind of doctor do I need to see?" Although your internist may be able to give you a fairly reliable diagnosis of IBS, it would be a good idea to consult with a gastroenterologist. Gastroenterologists are physicians who specialize in treating disorders of the intestinal tract. As specialists, they will be the most knowledgeable about IBS. They will know what to look for to rule out other possible causes for your symptoms. They are also your best source for the most helpful, up-to-date information on your condition.

How to Find a Doctor

Word of mouth and personal recommendations are always your best bet. If not, your physician can usually steer you in the right direction.

View your initial consultation somewhat like a job interview. On a job interview, you are not just selling yourself, but assessing whether or not you would be happy working in that environment. In the doctor's office, evaluate your comfort level. Is the office clean and well maintained? Is the office staff courteous and helpful? How long was the wait time for your appointment? Is this wait time typical for this office? Be in touch with your tolerance level on this subject. If you are quite pleased with your doctor, you may find them to be worth the wait. On the other hand, some people absolutely detest being kept waiting. If you fall into that category, the stress of the waiting room might outweigh the doctor's positive attributes and you might be better served elsewhere.

How comfortable do you feel with the doctor? Do you feel as if the doctor is concerned with your welfare? Are they responsive to your concerns and questions? Do you feel rushed or do you think that the doctor will take the time to meet your needs? Again, you want to make sure that you have found a person that you feel you can work well with.

Catherine, a thirty-four-year-old legal secretary, struck pay dirt with the first person she went to see, a gastroenterologist recommended by a coworker. "I love my doctor! Even though he's young, he really seems to know what he's talking about. He takes the time to listen to me and never makes me feel like I'm just being a crybaby. He works with me like we're a team in dealing with my problem. Feeling like I have a say in what happens to me has really helped me to regain a sense of control over my illness *and* my life."

Given the socially sensitive nature of the symptoms of IBS you need a doctor with whom you can openly discuss your discomforts without excessive embarrassment or the dangerous alternative of withholding information. If you feel rushed, intimidated, or worried that the doctor is not really listening to you, express this to the doctor. If you aren't satisfied with their response, you might want to think about consulting with someone else.

What Your Doctor Can Do

You must also have reasonable expectations about what your doctor can do for you. IBS, unfortunately, is a chronic condition, marked by episodes of exacerbation and periods of remission. Therefore, your doctor cannot cure you. They can, however, work to ensure an accurate diagnosis, help you to identify triggers, and provide you with a treatment plan for symptomatic relief.

Remember that most doctors have very busy practices, and their tight appointment schedule can be thrown off by emergencies, phone calls, or a late arrival from their hospital rounds. Therefore, once you have an ongoing relationship with a gastroenterologist, be patient with them. You never know when you may be the one who is requiring extra time and attention.

You can help maximize your time with your doctor by being organized about your symptoms and concerns. It's always a good idea to write these down ahead of time and bring them with you to your appointment. This allows your doctor to quickly get a sense of where your discomforts and anxieties lie and thus give you the answers and reassurance that you are seeking.

It is quite common to become overwhelmed and to have difficulty taking in all of the information given to you during an office visit. Sometimes, all you need to do is write your questions down and save them for the next visit. Other times, uncertainty or falsely remembered information can cause a lot of distress. Under these circumstances, it is okay to call your doctor if you have a legitimate question. Don't put yourself through unnecessary torment just because you don't want to be a bother.

Be Your Own Advocate

No pun intended, but listen to your gut. If something your doctor is telling you isn't sitting right with you, by all means, speak up! If you don't understand or agree with what your doctor is saying, say so. You have the right to be an active participant in your health care.

It can be difficult to assert yourself to a doctor. They represent an authority figure and you are, in a sense, dependent on them. This feeling of vulnerability and the need to show respect may make you hesitant about standing up for yourself. However, doctors are only human, and no one knows your body as well as you do, so it is important that you advocate for yourself when necessary.

Now, I teach assertiveness for a living, so you might be surprised to hear about the difficulty I had recently in dealing with a doctor. This physician had recommended that a diagnostic procedure be performed on my young son. Every time my son had undergone this particular procedure, the results had come up negative. The doctor's rationale for repeating the test didn't really make sense to me. The test was somewhat of an ordeal in that my son had to be sedated, which involved a period of fasting and two shots, one in each leg, which, to a five-year-old, can be quite traumatic. Since, to my mind, the test had not produced any significant results in the past, I refused to consent to the procedure.

The doctor grew quite angry. As he examined my son, he did not respond at all to my son's attempts to engage him in conversation. A part of me was very upset with this doctor for taking his feelings out on my son. But the unhealthy part of me had an extremely difficult time tolerating the fact that this doctor was mad at me. I had to keep telling myself, "You can do this. You can keep your mouth shut and not give in to this person just because you don't like anybody to be mad at you. Spending ten minutes more with this person is much better than putting my little guy through such a terrible ordeal." Afterward, I was glad that I had stuck to my guns. I eventually found an option where the test could be performed without sedation. But if I hadn't protested, this doctor would never have made that option available to us. Although it isn't always easy, self-advocacy can be crucial.

Stand Up and Say It

A quick little assertiveness lesson here may help—and you'll find a more in-depth discussion in chapter 9. Assertion involves identifying and expressing your rights, feelings, and preferences. Sometimes, it's just helpful to say "ouch," even if it changes nothing. Good assertiveness maximizes the probability of having a successful resolution of the problem with another person because it is designed to minimize defensiveness on their part.

The simplest thing to remember about being assertive is to use I-statements. This means that you say what you have to say by talking about how you *feel* about what the other person did, as in "I was very unhappy when you did such and such" or "I would really prefer it if you would talk to me in a calmer manner." The advantage of this is that you're talking about your perspective on the problem, as opposed to lambasting the other person for screwing up. The minute you say to someone "You did this," whatever "this" may be, you automatically put them on the defensive. They are forced to explain and defend their actions, rather than focusing on trying to resolve the conflict. When you use an I-statement, you are giving the other person a way to save face because you aren't judging their actions—you're merely stating how their actions made you feel. You are therefore taking some responsibility for the role that you play in the dispute. Unfortunately, this doesn't mean that this is how the other person is going to perceive your statement. Some people will respond with defensiveness or hostility no matter how nicely you put things.

So, to forge a good working relationship with your doctor, you can say things like "I am very concerned about . . ." or "That doesn't sit right with me; can you explain it further?" Other good examples include "I'm not sure I am understanding you correctly" and "I'm frustrated by the fact that I am still feeling so bad, what can we do about it?" Again, you want to feel free to discuss your concerns, but to do so in a spirit of cooperation.

The First Visit

If you have already been to the doctor, you can skip this section or use it as a review to better understand what went on. During your first appointment, you doctor will most likely take a detailed history. They will want to hear about how you have been feeling and will ask about other symptoms that you might be experiencing in order to rule out other disorders. They will ask when your symptoms first appeared and about factors that may be contributing to your distress, such as stress, use of laxatives and other medications, and any history of food intolerance. They will ask about risk factors and family history. You can help to use your time with the doctor most efficiently by having your information organized ahead of time. It would be helpful to write up a brief list of your symptoms as well as your questions and concerns. Ask family members about their health history and that of the extended family. The more you know, the greater a help you will be.

After gathering some background information, your physician will conduct a routine physical examination. If the problem is irritable bowel, your physical exam will probably be normal, except for, perhaps, some tenderness on the lower left side of your abdomen. Quick, a pop quiz! What's down there? Your sigmoid colon, did you remember that? The sigmoid colon sometimes becomes sore from the muscle spasms that are so common in IBS.

Following the physical examination, your doctor will outline a series of tests. They will explain to you what the tests entail and what information is being sought. The doctor should be able to give you some indication of what possible diagnoses are being considered. At this point, your doctor may even be able to initiate a discussion of treatment options.

Diagnostic Tests

Irritable bowel syndrome used to be considered a diagnosis of exclusion, which means that IBS was diagnosed after everything else was ruled out. In other words, "If it's not this, that, or the other thing, well I guess it must be IBS." It is now thought that IBS can be positively diagnosed based on the symptom picture. The criteria can be summarized as abdominal pain relieved by defecation and a change in the frequency and consistency of stools for at least a three-month period. Based on the symptoms, a diagnosis of irritable bowel syndrome can be made with confidence. In most cases, therefore, diagnostic testing can be kept to a minimum. You can rest assured that it's very unlikely that other, more serious disorders will be missed. Further testing would definitely be indicated if your symptom picture included anemia, bleeding from the rectum or in the stool, fever, significant weight loss, or sudden onset of symptoms after age forty.

Basic Tests

A fairly likely test scenario would start with a blood test in order to check for iron deficiency which could be caused by internal bleeding. A stool sample would also be taken, looking for blood in the stool, again to rule out intestinal bleeding. Intestinal bleeding is not a symptom of IBS. Thus, any sign of intestinal bleeding would indicate a different diagnosis and warrant further testing. Don't be alarmed if you've seen some blood after using the bathroom. Bright red blood on the outside of the stool is most likely the result of a hemorrhoid or a fissure, which is a crack in the lining of the anus. Do tell your doctor if this has happened to you.

There is some disagreement among members of the medical community as to whether or not further, more invasive testing is necessary when the symptom picture seems to indicate irritable bowel syndrome. Many doctors believe that if there is no evidence of intestinal bleeding or symptoms associated with other digestive disorders, the diagnosis can be made without further testing. Other doctors may be more cautious and request further testing just to be on the safe side. The decision to undergo additional procedures should be made by you and your doctor. If you trust your doctor and their rationale makes sense to you, then go with their recommendations regarding diagnostic procedures. Further testing is always indicated if there is any sign or suspicion of intestinal bleeding.

Looking for Answers

Many patients with IBS are in so much pain and discomfort that they're convinced that something more serious is wrong with them, and thus want their doctors to keep performing tests until they find something definite. That was certainly true for Paula, a thirty-one-year-old office furniture salesperson, who came to see me because she was extremely concerned that her doctors had overlooked something. "I want them to do every test in the book on me until they find an answer. The tests keep coming back normal. They must be missing something! How can it be that the tests say that there's nothing wrong with me? I feel like I'm dying!" The thing that most people fear, of course, is cancer. Many people worry that the tests have missed it and that by the time the cancer is detected, it will be too late. Although these fears are very natural and certainly commonplace, you don't want to let fear overcome common sense. If you have no symptoms of colon cancer, and your doctor assures you that there are no signs of such, it would be foolish to put yourself through the anxiety, discomfort, and expense of unnecessary testing.

Sigmoidoscopy

What are some of these other tests? A relatively common procedure, often used when IBS is suspected, is the sigmoidoscopic examination. A sigmoidoscopy is a relatively noninvasive test (easy for me to say!) that your doctor might recommend. The procedure can be performed right in the doctor's office, as there is minimal preparation needed. The sigmoidoscope is a lighted instrument that passes through the rectum and allows your doctor to view the lower portion of the colon. The sigmoidoscopy helps your doctor to rule out a structural or infectious disease. If diarrhea is a predominant symptom, your doctor might do a colon biopsy to rule out colitis, an inflammation of the intestinal lining.

Barium Enema

If you are over the age of forty, or have a family history of colon cancer or polyps, your doctor may recommend a barium enema. Sounds ominous, huh? It's really not quite so bad. A barium enema is only a series of X-rays. The problem is that unlike X-rays on other parts of the body, preliminary preparation is necessary in order to make the digestive tract visible. For an upper GI series, in which pictures are taken of the stomach and small intestine, a special solution is given to the patient to drink. For the lower part of the digestive system, it is necessary for a barium enema to be administered so that pictures may be taken of the colon and rectum. You can see why you might want to avoid unnecessary testing!

Colonoscopy

A colonoscopy is another common diagnostic procedure for the intestinal tract, but it is not generally required when the diagnosis is irritable bowel syndrome. Your doctor might recommend a colonoscopy if you are over the age of fifty or there is a family history of colon cancer. A colonoscopy would also be recommended if there is any suspicion of cancer or polyps. A colonoscopy is similar to the sigmoidoscopy except that the tube is longer and therefore can be used to examine the entire colon. Unfortunately, this procedure requires that the colon be cleaned out. If your IBS is diarrhea-predominant, you probably feel as if your colon is cleaned out on a daily basis as it is! Regardless, you would be instructed to take laxatives on the day before or the morning of the test, which obviously would result in diarrhea-like symptoms. You would also be restricted to consuming clear liquids. Due to the discomfort of the exam, patients are generally given a sedative before the procedure begins. Although it may sound somewhat unpleasant, don't be afraid of this test. If there is any suspicion of cancer, it is essential that this test be performed. Colon cancer is extremely treatable if it is caught early. Don't let anxiety and procrastination put you on a road that you might not want to be on, namely battling a terminal illness.

What If It's Not IBS?

Here is another area where a little information can ease a lot of anxiety. Knowing the symptoms of other digestive disorders, can help you to accept the diagnosis of irritable bowel syndrome with confidence and calm your fears that the doctors have overlooked something more serious.

Inflammatory Bowel Diseases

The inflammatory bowel diseases, ulcerative colitis and Crohn's disease, are great examples of structural diseases (again, as opposed to functional diseases) because they involve inflammation of the lining of the digestive tract. Ulcerative colitis involves an inflammation in the lining of the colon. Rectal bleeding is a predominant symptom, as are frequent, urgent attacks of diarrhea. As opposed to IBS, these attacks are urgent enough to wake a person from sleep. Fatigue, fever, weight loss, and cramping are also seen in varying degrees.

Crohn's disease is considered to be the more serious of the two. In Crohn's disease, the inflammation can be found in all areas of the digestive tract, and most particularly in the small intestine and the colon. The inflammation can be so severe that it spreads to other organs, through connections called fistulas. Symptoms of Crohn's disease include diarrhea (with or without bleeding), abdominal cramps, anemia, weight loss, and fatigue.

Diverticular Disease

Another relatively common digestive disorder is diverticular disease. It is possible for IBS and diverticular disease to coexist. Diverticulosis refers to the formation of small pockets in the lining of the colon. These small sacs can become inflamed, often due to food, such as seeds, that becomes trapped. When this occurs, diverticulitis is diagnosed. Symptoms of diverticulitis are pain and fever, with possible nausea and vomiting.

Colon Cancer

And now, the one that you are probably most afraid of: the "Big C," colon cancer. Although many of the symptoms of colon cancer, such as persistent diarrhea, alternating diarrhea and constipation, and abdominal pain and cramping, are similar to irritable bowel syndrome, there are some important differences. Blood in the stool is a significant sign of the presence of colon cancer. Abdominal pain and cramping are not necessarily relieved by defecation, as is the case in IBS. Loss of weight, poor appetite, and fatigue are also symptomatic of cancer. Keeping in mind these very important differences will help you stay much calmer as you cope with your distressing symptoms. Knowing the difference between the symptoms of IBS and colon cancer can go a long way to reassure you that you aren't dying, even when you're feeling so sick that you can't even leave your house. Your faith in your doctor and their diagnosis will ultimately put your fears to rest.

The Good News

Now that you have read about some of the other scary things that can go wrong with your digestive system, here is some good news. A diagnosis of IBS means that there is no need for surgery. IBS does not involve a shorter life expectancy. Lastly, IBS has not been shown to lead to other, more serious disorders. You may be quite relieved to hear this, as this is a very common concern of many IBS patients. Susan, a hardworking office manager, expressed this fear: "I kept worrying about the damage that all this sickness was doing to my body. During bouts of diarrhea, which seemed constant, I could barely eat. I kept thinking that I was going to end up with something more serious, either because of a lack of vitamins or damage to my body from being so sick all the time. I felt so much better when I realized that that was not the case."

Exercise: A Self-Help Souvenir

The worksheet below is designed to help to reduce unnecessary anxiety regarding being correctly diagnosed. As a reward for all of your hard work to date, I have filled part of this one in for you. Xerox the worksheet and place in in your wallet, on your refrigerator, or next to your toilet. Just make sure it is handy wherever you are likely to be when you are obsessively worrying. Add to the worksheet anything that you think might be helpful to keep you sane, even when you are feeling so sick that you are sure you must only have a short time left on earth.

I Do Not Have Cancer!

Fear	Logic
I'm dying!	My doctor says I don't have cancer.
It *must* be cancer.	I don't have the symptoms of colon cancer.
My doctor must not know what he or she is talking about.	Based on my symptoms, my doctor can tell that I have an irritable bowel.
I can't handle this!	Although this isn't easy, I can learn to manage my IBS and have a good life.

What Treatments Are Available?

Now that you know how a diagnosis of irritable bowel syndrome is made, you might be wondering what your physican can do to help you feel better. Although they can't cure your IBS, they can offer symptomatic relief and recommend lifestyle changes for better management of the disorder.

Dietary Changes

The first thing your doctor may do is take a look at your diet to identify anything that might be triggering your symptoms, and then suggest changes. Likely culprits are laxatives, alcohol, sorbitol, and lactose. Your doctor may perform a lactose-intolerance test and prescribe a reduced lactose diet.

Medication

Your doctor may recommend medication. This might be an over-the-counter product or something only available by prescription. Your understanding of the way that your digestive system is supposed to work will take the mystery out of any recommended medication, again helping you to regain that all-important feeling of control.

If your predominant symptom is constipation, it is highly likely that your doctor will recommend an over-the-counter psyllium bulking agent. As their name implies, these agents add bulk to the stool, which helps it move through the system at a steady pace. Don't use any of the over-the-counter nonbulking laxatives. Chronic use of laxatives will exacerbate your condition and may lead to permanent malfunctioning of your colon.

For the treatment of diarrhea, your doctor may recommend a nonprescription antidiarrheal agent. This type of agent works by increasing the absorption of water from fecal matter, slowing intestinal contractions and transit time, and strengthening the sphincter control of the rectum. It is extremely important that you use any over-the-counter medications only with the blessing of your doctor.

Some medications available only by prescription are used to treat certain IBS symptoms. Your doctor might prescribe an antispasmodic, which, as its name implies, reduces intestinal spasms. Reducing these spasms results in less pain, cramping, and diarrhea.

When abdominal pain is severe, an antidepressant medication may be prescribed. This class of medication has been shown to have a pain-reducing effect, by acting on the areas of the brain that are involved in pain perception. One of the side effects of antidepressants can be constipation, so it is probably better suited for patients whose IBS is diarrhea-predominant.

Your doctor may recommend an antidepressant or antianxiety medication if they believe that you are also experiencing a coexisting anxiety or depressive disorder. If your doctor believes that you should be taking one of these psychotropic medications, I would strongly urge you to consult with a psychiatrist, who specializes in the pharmacological treatment of psychiatric symptoms.

Other Treatments

Other forms of treatment have been found to be effective in reducing the distress of IBS. The advantage of nondrug treatment is that you don't have to worry about unpleasant side effects and you will learn skills that can be used in the future, whenever you experience an exacerbation of your condition. Psychotherapy and specialized techniques, such as biofeedback, relaxation training, and hypnotherapy, have been shown to reduce IBS symptoms. Please feel free to discuss any of these options with your doctor.

Prognosis

Although IBS has a chronic course, with periods of exacerbation and periods of remission, treatment has been shown to be effective in limiting the duration of the illness, reducing the frequency of outbreaks and lessening the severity of symptoms. One study of a large group of IBS patients (Harvey, Mauad, and Brown 1987) found that providing patients with education about the syndrome, combined with the use of a high-fiber diet, and in some cases, short-term use of antispasmodic medication, resulted in significant symptom improvement within six months. They checked in with these people five years later and found that two-thirds of them were virtually symptom-free. Wouldn't you like to find yourself in that category?

Setting Your Course

You can now consider yourself a well-informed patient. Take a moment to congratulate yourself. The material that you have just successfully taken in is complex, and you are now ready to become an active participant in your medical treatment. Like the sailboat captain, you can use your doctor to provide you with valuable information toward the goal of feeling healthy. The rest is up to you.

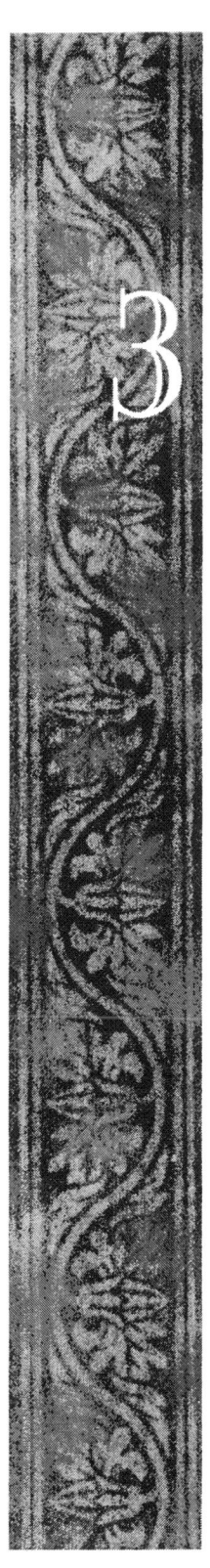

3 FOOD IS NOT THE ENEMY!

In many cultures the preparation and enjoyment of food make up the centerpiece of a reassuring, comforting social experience. However, in our society of fast food and the often unreasonable quest for a thin waistline, the pleasure of mealtime is all too frequently overshadowed by pressure, guilt, and deprivation. Worse yet, if you are a person suffering from IBS, mealtimes may also be fraught with terror!

Detective Work

One of your first lines of defense against this disorder is to take a good look at your eating habits. Don't panic: you aren't going to be condemned to a permanent diet of tea and toast. Although it is true that certain foods can trigger or exacerbate IBS symptoms, with a little knowledge, research, and planning, you can discover which foods are helpful and which are best avoided. In addition, taking a few simple steps to make your mealtimes more relaxing and pleasurable will also help to reduce your IBS symptoms. Remember that eating in a more healthful manner will not just help you to start to better manage your IBS, but will also help to reduce your chances of other diseases and go a long way toward improved mental health.

It will take a little effort on your part to determine the effect that various foods have on your system, but it will be well worth it. It will be your job to uncover the relationship between certain types of food and *your* intestinal difficulties.

Exercise: The Food Diary

In order to uncover the relationship between food and physical symptoms, you will need to keep track of what you eat and how you feel. Take a look at the worksheet on the next page. You can make copies of the worksheet or buy a small notebook and copy the headings.

Filling out the diary is really quite simple. Just write down what you have eaten and what symptoms you are experiencing. Try to keep your notebook or your worksheets handy so you can fill them in in a timely manner. Memories tend to be quite unreliable, particularly when it comes to food.

Write down the time you experience symptoms, even if you cannot necessarily connect them with a meal or snack. Your symptom list could consist of things such as abdominal pain or cramps, diarrhea, constipation, bloating, and/or excessive gas. Other symptoms might be nausea, belching, heartburn, or lack of appetite. When possible, try to categorize your symptoms on a severity scale of 1 to 5, with 1 reflecting a mild discomfort and 5 representing severe distress. The severity rating scale will not only serve to give you information regarding your current symptoms, but will also provide you with some concrete feedback when you are starting to feel better and your symptoms diminish.

Food Diary

Date _____ Severity—1 (low) to 5 (high)

Time	Food Eaten	Symptoms

How the Food Diary Works

Keep an active food diary for at least three weeks. This time frame will give you a pretty good picture of your food choices and your physical response. Down the road, should you experience an IBS relapse or flare-up, it might be a good idea to repeat the food diary process to see if there has been any change in your eating habits or your body's reaction.

People always ask me what they should eat while keeping a food diary. "Should I only eat all of the so-called right foods, or should I eat the foods that I think make me sick just to find out for sure?" Well, doesn't it seem crazy to eat foods that you know will cause you distress? The whole idea of treatment is to feel better! The information in this chapter will help guide you toward healthy food choices. Experimenting is fine, as long as the conditions are right, e.g. stressors are low, you are feeling fairly calm, or you are in a position to handle any potential negative consequences because you don't have any pressing social commitments and can be home.

Do not become overly restrictive with your diet without the approval of your doctor and the supervision of a registered dietitian. An exclusionary diet can be dangerous due to the risk of depletion of essential nutrients. If you don't feel that you can maintain a balanced, healthy food plan that is least offensive to your system on your own, a consultation with a nutritionist would be a good idea.

Before branding a food as troublesome, it is important to make sure that your symptoms are not simply due to eating a meal that is too heavy. When we eat a meal, intestinal activity is increased, a response called the gastrocolic reflex. A meal that is large and calorie-laden may exaggerate this response, resulting in abdominal pain, cramping, and diarrhea. Keep this reflex in mind as you evaluate the relationship between the foods you eat and your subsequent symptoms. If you suspect a particular food is problematic for your system, you may want to try it in a smaller portion and as part of a lighter meal and see what happens.

Is It Worth the Trouble?

If this sounds like too much work, don't forget what a drag it is to be chained to a bathroom. A few weeks' worth of vigilance can give you vital information for reducing your symptoms and freeing you up to enjoy life. Greg's experience is a good example. When Greg first came to see me, he was very angry about the way that IBS was affecting his life. He had recently graduated from college and was actively looking for a job, but his attacks of diarrhea had really shaken his confidence about setting up interviews with potential employers. When I asked him to keep a food diary, his frustrations all came pouring out. "You don't understand. I *need* to get a job. I'm so sick of reading the want ads, writing cover letters, and sending out résumés. Now you want me to write down everything I eat. You have got to be kidding. I just want my old life back. I want to be normal."

With encouragement, Greg did finally agree to keep track of what he ate and how he felt. It didn't take him long to realize that his typical fast-food lunch of hamburgers and french fries was contributing to considerable distress during afternoon job interviews. Seeing this connection spelled out clearly on his worksheet helped him to plan things differently. When possible, he scheduled interviews for the morning after a light breakfast of bran cereal. He found that this generally helped to keep his colon quiet. As he was only twenty-two, he wasn't quite ready to give up on McDonald's altogether, so he would indulge himself on the weekends when he was feeling less pressured. Becoming an expert on your own personal relationship with food can really help you to regain a feeling of control over your life.

Look Out for Pitfalls

Greg's story also illustrates the point that just because you identify a certain food as being troublesome for your system, it doesn't mean that you can never have that food again. Watch out for black-and-white labeling of food. Dieters frequently make this mistake, branding food as good or bad. I'll hear them say, "I have been very bad. I had sugar today." I'll ask them, "Sugar? Was it sugar in an apple? Was it sugar in a fig bar, or was it sugar in a piece of chocolate cake?" The point is that no food is inherently good or bad. Some foods are healthier because of a higher nutrient content, while others offer little in terms of fueling our bodies. The problem with this type of black-and-white labeling is that people tend to feel hopeless or self-critical after they have given in to temptation and eaten something that they consider to be forbidden. These negative feelings then leave the person at high risk for giving up on trying to eat healthy, thus creating a negative cycle of self-destruction.

IBS patients are also at risk for this type of food labeling. You may brand certain foods as deadly and always to be avoided. While it is a good idea to try to avoid eating foods that you know are upsetting to your system, complete blacklisting of food has several potential negative side effects. The first is that you could become filled with resentment and self-pity. "How come the rest of the world can sit around at a party chowing down on nacho dip, while I'm stuck nibbling on a piece of celery?" This kind of "poor me" thinking rarely leads to good self-care or good social functioning.

The second potential pitfall of negative food labeling is that you might panic after eating something from your Forbidden Foods list. Say you decide to reach for a piece of that fried shrimp that's being passed around at the annual company party. You then become hypervigilant about the effect this is going to have on your system. You become distracted from the conversation around you as you begin to focus on any little intestinal twinge. Your anxiety begins to rise, thus triggering the kind of gut reaction that you have been fearing. You can see how easy it can be to work yourself into some kind of a state.

Greg's story shows that so-called troublesome foods can sometimes be enjoyed if the conditions are favorable. The whole point is to identify which foods are friendly and which foods are potential triggers. This information can help you to plan for healthy food choices so that you feel in control of your life rather than feeling controlled by your colon.

Common Culprits

Scientists have identified some foods that appear to be particularly troublesome for IBS patients. You may have even seen some lists of such foods. I don't know about you, but every time I read one of these lists, my eyes glaze over. It's hard to remember which foods are known to be helpful and which foods are considered to be more harmful. One way to try to retain this information is to understand *why* certain foods trigger IBS symptoms. As you read through the following sections, keep in mind our previous discussion of the digestive system. It will help you to visualize and make sense of the information that will be presented.

Common sense will also lead you to healthy food choices. You already know which foods have a reputation for irritating the intestines, particularly spicy or gassy foods. You also probably have some sense of the foods that cause difficulty for your system. These are the foods to avoid when you are under stress or when experiencing an IBS flare-up. You can slowly reintroduce these foods when you are feeling better.

Vegetables

All your life you have been told "Eat your vegetables! They're good for you." For the most part, this is true. Vegetables are a good source of fiber, which serves to bulk up your stool (are you visualizing this?) and helps to regulate your system. However, some vegetables are gas-producing and contribute to pain, bloating, and flatulence. These are often the ones you hear jokes about. As a child I remember my mother refusing to serve baked beans due to the chorus of "Beans, beans, the musical fruit" that was inevitable. Similarly, while working as a waitress while still in high school, I was quite taken aback when a customer requested carrots and "gas balls" to go with his roast beef. He was referring to brussels sprouts.

Troublesome vegetables generally fall into two categories. The first are members of the legume family, namely beans and lentils. The second notorious crime family is made up of the head vegetables, such as cabbage, broccoli, and cauliflower. Onions may also be problematic for some people. As you review your food diary, look to see if you have eaten any of these vegetables and check to see what effect, if any, they had on your system.

Sugars and Artificial Sweeteners

Like vegetables, some other foods that you perceive as healthy might in actuality be troublesome. Fruits and many low-cal diet products fit into this category. You may not think of fruits as containing sugar, but they do—a type of sugar called fructose. Fructose is poorly absorbed by the small intestine, as is sorbitol, a sweetener used in many diet foods and chewing gums. You may remember that it is the small intestine's job to absorb nutrients into the bloodstream. As fructose and sorbitol are not well absorbed by the small intestine, they enter the colon, where they are attacked by bacteria. This results in excessive gas, bloating, and possibly diarrhea.

Look at your food diary. Have any of your symptoms been triggered by certain kinds of fruit or fruit juice? If so, which kinds? Citrus fruits (oranges, lemons, and limes) have been known to aggravate an irritable bowel.

But don't throw the baby out with the bathwater. Fruits have a high fiber content, and fiber is quite beneficial for IBS patients. Some fruits have a reputation for being especially well suited to IBS sufferers, particularly apples, pears, and bananas. It's important to learn how your own body reacts to a particular food so that you can make an informed choice for yourself. In addition to being an excellent source of fiber, fruits are loaded with many essential nutrients and should therefore make up a large portion of your diet.

Also review your food diary to ascertain a reactivity to diet products or diet soda. If you believe a relationship exists, you would be wise to avoid these foods and find other ways to reduce your caloric intake.

A third sugar that causes much the same difficulty as fructose and sorbitol is lactose, a sugar found in milk and dairy products. In fact, it is estimated that up to 40 percent of IBS patients are lactose intolerant. The condition is caused by a deficit in the enzyme lactase, which is needed for the digestion of lactose. When lactose is undigested, this milk sugar ferments in the colon, as a result of being set upon by colon bacteria, again causing gas, bloating, and diarrhea.

As 40 percent is a fairly significant number, it would be a good idea to rule out lactose intolerance as a cause for your symptoms. Check your food diary. Do you experience diarrhea and bloating two hours after eating a meal that contained a high amount of milk or other dairy products? If so, discuss the possibility of lactose intolerance with your doctor. They may perform a lactose breath tolerance test or recommend adherence to a two- to three-week lactose-free diet. This would involve avoiding cheese, milk, and baked goods. Again, this type of restrictive diet should only be undertaken under the supervision of a physician.

Unfortunately, identifying a lactose intolerance might not necessarily mean that you're out of the woods. DiPalma and colleagues (1994) looked at the relationship between an identified lactose intolerance and IBS symptoms. They found that although lactose intolerance certainly contributed to intestinal symptoms, diagnosing the problem did not cause a significant decrease in those symptoms. This is probably because other factors contributed to the irritable bowel condition. The main advantage of identifying a lactose intolerance was that it helped patients to be more aware of the relationship between food and physical symptoms.

If you find that you are lactose intolerant, it is essential that you obtain the proper amount of calcium, as avoidance of dairy products leaves you at risk for calcium deficiency. Your doctor may recommend that you take a lactase supplement to help your body absorb the lactose. Also keep in mind that people with lactose intolerance can tolerate up to one cup of milk a day. Cheese, yogurt, and ice cream may be tolerated as well, because they have less lactose. Lactose-free milk is also available. In addition, your doctor may recommend, particularly if you are female, that you take a calcium supplement.

Wheat Products

Like fruits and vegetables, wheat products may serve as a double-edged sword for some IBS patients. The good guys are unrefined carbohydrates, found in whole-wheat breads, cereals, pasta, and rice, again due to their high fiber content.

Refined carbohydrates, the ones found in white bread, white flour, and white rice, are probably best avoided. Besides offering little in the way of nutrients and fiber, they reduce the bulk of the stool. This may result in intense muscle spasms, causing pain and diarrhea. The typical American diet tends to be overly high in refined carbohydrates. Your food diary tells all. Do you eat like a typical American? Keep in mind the effect that these substances have on your body and you will find it easier to make better food choices.

Fats

Of course, you already know that fatty foods aren't good for you. But, damn, they taste good! Well, here's more bad news. Fat, found in fried food, gravies, cream sauces, and ice cream, is very bad for IBS sufferers. When fatty foods enter the digestive system, a hormone called CCK (cholecystokinin) is released. This same hormone is responsible for stimulating colonic contractions, so it's easy to see why it is believed that eating fatty foods stimulates strong contractions that result in abdominal pain, cramping, and diarrhea. Check your food diary. Have you been indulging? Do you pay for it later?

Other Irritants

Limiting the amount of alcohol and caffeine you ingest is always good advice. This seems to be especially true for IBS, as both are known to irritate the system. Caffeine can stimulate colon contractions, and you know what that means, right? Alcohol, particularly red wine, can also upset your system. Avoiding these substances when you are feeling ill, or cutting them out altogether, is probably a very good idea.

Friendly Foods

So, what's left to eat? Before you get too discouraged, please keep in mind that everybody is different. Just because your best friend finds broccoli to be deadly for her system doesn't mean that it will have the same effect on you. Remember that your own body is going to react differently at different times, because hormones and stress are also triggers for IBS symptoms. At certain times, you will find that you're more symptomatic regardless of what you eat. Thus, a fair evaluation of any food can only be made when other factors can be ruled out.

Did your mother ever recommend the soothing, bland BRAT diet when you had diarrhea as a child? This stands for bananas, rice, applesauce, and toast. This advice is still quite sound. If you substitute whole wheat toast and brown rice, then all of the foods on the list are good sources of fiber and are usually well tolerated. For the most part, it appears that fiber is your colon's best friend. Of course, nothing in life is quite so simple. Read on.

Fiber: The Good, the Bad, and the Confusing

There is ample evidence that a high-fiber, low-fat diet is your best bet for physical health and your best guard against disease. Your newly acquired expertise regarding how the digestive system works will serve you well as you begin to understand why this is so.

Fiber is known as a good guy because it gives a heavier mass to stools. This bulking effect helps the stool to move more quickly and easily through your large intestine, as well as helping you to easily eliminate the stool. One of the advantages of fiber for IBS sufferers is that the quicker transit time leaves less time for your body to react to irritants.

Though it might seem counterintuitive, the effect of fiber on intestinal speed is a positive one for both diarrhea and constipation. For people who suffer from constipation, the increase in fiber helps to soften the stool and bulk it up so that it moves along more quickly. For diarrhea sufferers, the bulking effect helps to slow down the excessive speed and firm up the loose, watery stools that are characteristic of diarrhea.

Soluble versus Insoluble

You may have heard the terms soluble and insoluble fiber; understanding the distinction is helpful in combating IBS symptoms. Soluble fiber forms a gel when it meets up with water. Foods high in soluble fiber are recommended for diarrhea because the soluble fiber adds substance to the stool. Examples of foods high in soluble fiber include beans, fruits, oats, and barley. If your food diary indicates that your IBS tends to be diarrhea-predominant, you might want to try including more of these foods in your diet.

Insoluble fiber does not dissolve in water. Thus, it helps to retain water in your stool. As you already know, this softens the stool, helps it to retain bulk, and allows it to move along and out more quickly. Insoluble fiber is found in wheat bran, whole grains, and many vegetables. If constipation is the predominant way that your IBS manifests itself, add more of these foods and evaluate the results.

Bran: Friend or Foe?

A quick word about bran. When doctors were first reporting the health benefits of a high-fiber diet, bran became all the rage. Had you even heard of a bran muffin twenty years ago? Bran is generally recommended to IBS patients to alleviate constipation because it softens and bulks the stool, making it easier to eliminate and thereby reducing straining.

An interesting study was performed by Francis and Whorwell (1994), who theorized that bran actually worsens IBS symptoms. They looked at the response of individuals to various types of fiber, including bran. Within their group of subjects, 55 percent reported that bran worsened their symptoms, with only 10 percent reporting improvement. Other sources of fiber appeared to have a more neutral effect. As this is only one study, and it was based upon self-report, it can't be definitively stated that bran should be taboo for IBS patients. But this study does point to the need for you to become your very own research scientist and make a careful assessment of the effects that certain foods have on your individual body. If your food diary indicates that your system has difficulty tolerating **bran**, try to get your fiber from other food sources or a psyllium fiber supplement.

Tips and Tricks

Don't say that I didn't warn you that this could get confusing. Just remember: The most important thing is not to be afraid of fiber. Many people are very hesitant about adding fiber to their diets, because they have been so traumatized by painful or distressing IBS symptoms that they're afraid that fiber will make it worse. I've heard it both ways. "Oh, no. Every time I eat more fiber I get constipated." "What, are you crazy? If I eat more fiber, I just know I'll get the runs." This is why your food diary is so important. You now know that you may be reacting to foods high in fiber for other reasons, e.g. the fructose in fruits, the gas-producing tendencies of some vegetables, or perhaps a bran intolerance. Figure out which fiber sources are easier on your system. Determine whether you need more soluble or insoluble fiber based on your predominant symptoms. Make your food choices accordingly and evaluate the results.

Be prepared. Sometimes adding fiber to your system can cause a temporary increase in symptoms before it begins to help. One way to counteract this is to add fiber slowly, giving your body time to adjust. You might find it preferable to start with a psyllium fiber supplement and then slowly introduce food fiber. Drink plenty of water, which works with the fiber to add bulk. So, fiber is good, bran may or may not be helpful, and get to know your own body. Got it?

Getting Personal

Trying to remember all of the above information can be quite a daunting task. Which foods are helpful? Which ones should you avoid? Many of my patients have found it extremely helpful to make up their own personal food guide.

Exercise: Your Personal Food Guide

After about three weeks of keeping your food diary, you should have enough information to identify which foods are friendly to your system and which foods are troublesome. As you can see by the worksheet below, that's all you need to know.

Take a good look at your food diary. Identify those foods that appear to exacerbate your symptoms, and write them down under the heading Troublesome Foods. You may see that many of these foods fall into the categories that we discussed earlier. Go through your diary again, identify the foods that appear safe, and list them under the Friendly Foods column.

If you're unsure about a certain food, list it with a question mark following it. Eliminate it from your diet for a few days and look for symptom improvement. Gradually reintroduce the food during periods when your IBS seems to have gone into remission, then evaluate your ability to tolerate it. You may find that you can tolerate a certain food in small doses or at certain times. Although you may need to repeat the test process a few times, you might find that a food you thought was forbidden can be safely enjoyed after all.

Personal Food Guide

Troublesome Foods   Friendly Foods

Looking for Patterns

To illustrate the benefit of drawing up your own personal food guide, let me show you the food guide filled out by a patient of mine, a young woman named Julie who worked as a flight attendant. If you have ever been in an airplane bathroom, you can imagine how distressing IBS was for Julie.

Julie's Food Guide

Troublesome Foods	Friendly Foods
Bagels	Yogurt
Bacon	Apples
Pears	Bananas
French fries	Brown rice
Gravy	Bran cereal
Tomato sauce	Chicken
Onions	Peas
Roasted red peppers	Baked potatoes
Diet soda	

Let's take a look at Julie's food guide and look for patterns. As none of the items on Julie's troublesome list are dairy products, there does not appear to be any evidence of lactose intolerance. She does seem to have difficulty with fatty foods and certain kinds of vegetables. Her difficulty with pears is surprising because many people find pears to have a helpful effect. Her Friendly Foods list contains a lot of foods with a high fiber content, which is good, and she doesn't appear to have a negative reaction to bran. Julie said that devising the list has really simplified the process of making helpful food choices. She has found that narrowing down the culprits and knowing which foods are safe has helped her tremendously, especially when her IBS flares up.

Use the same process to look for patterns in your personal food guide. Is there evidence of lactose intolerance? Do you have difficulties with bran, fats, diet foods, or certain kinds of fruits or vegetables? Does your Friendly Foods list contain fiber sources? Do you do better with soluble or insoluble fiber? You'll find that this type of organization and identification of patterns makes it much easier for you to figure out what to eat. Make sure to update your list as necessary. As you begin to feel better, you will see that all of your hard work has really paid off.

Healthy Choices, Healthy Living

As you work to change your eating habits so as to reduce your intestinal distress, it may also be a good time to incorporate other healthy eating strategies. You want to consider the nutritional values of the foods you eat, not just their calorie count. Strive for balance. Eat lots of naturally colorful food, which tends to be high in nutrients. The foods that are helpful for IBS are foods that are good for you in general. If one of the side effects of your IBS is that you eat in a more healthy manner, you have done a terrific job of turning adversity to your advantage.

One of the most helpful eating strategies is so simple that it's amazing that most people rarely think of it. Several years ago, I read of a study (Craighead and Allen 1995) in which patients with a history of problematic binge eating were given appetite awareness training. Their suggestions are quite applicable to anyone, binge eater or not. This training involves evaluating how hungry you are before eating and how sated you are after eating. Brilliant, huh? Before deciding what to eat, ask yourself, "How hungry am I?" Plan your meal or snack accordingly. After eating, wait a short while and then ask yourself, "Do I feel full?" before helping yourself to seconds.

Most adults have lost touch with their inner appetite controls, but children tend to be quite good at this. They excel at self-regulation if they aren't overly pressured by adults. Unfortunately, years of exposure to social pressure, self-imposed deprivation due to dieting, and binge eating have left some people without any clue as to their fuel needs. Internal cues of hunger and satiety get lost in the process. With practice, these internal sensations can be heard again.

Picking and Choosing

In addition to getting in touch with your hunger/satiety feelings, think about food preferences as you decide what to eat. Now you might say, "Oh, that's easy. I *prefer* to eat a large bowl of ice cream." While it is easy to be led astray by food preferences, you don't want to disregard them altogether. Weigh your options with a focus on nutritional value, but also ask yourself what you prefer. If you consistently ignore your food preferences, feelings of deprivation may arise, leaving you vulnerable to unhealthy binges. A meal or snack should leave you feeling satisfied, because that's an important part of feeling sated.

So, as you plan a meal or place your order in a restaurant, consider the following factors. How hungry are you? Which foods will sit best with your system? Which foods pack the best nutritional punch? What appeals to you? This quick analysis will be of tremendous help to you in making wise, healthy food choices.

If, after all this hard work, you're still confused or lack confidence in your ability to maintain a healthy food plan, you might want to consider consulting with a registered dietitian. You can ask your physician for a referral or call the American Dietetic Association for a list of local dietitians. Prior to making an appointment, make sure that the dietitian is familiar with irritable bowel syndrome and has a good understanding of the kinds of foods that you need to help to reduce symptoms but still ensure an adequate amount of required nutrients.

Making Mealtimes Merry

It is well known that external cues associated with a trauma can by themselves incite an anxiety reaction. War veterans become filled with terror when exposed to sudden loud noises such as fireworks. Although not quite as extreme, IBS distress can be traumatic. Since food can be a primary trigger for symptoms, anything associated with food can cause anxiety. Meals are no exception. They become events to be dreaded rather than enjoyable experiences.

Ann Marie's anxiety associated with meals led her to make a drastic decision. When she first came to see me, she was twenty-six years old, single, and working as an adminstrative assistant for a large manufacturing company. Ann Marie had had a couple of bad experiences where she got sick following meals out in restaurants with a date. Because these experiences were so stressful, Ann Marie had decided to stop dating altogether. She explained the rationale for this decision, "Last week, I went on a first date with a guy who seemed really nice. He took me to a beautiful restaurant, but it turned into a nightmare. I was barely through my entree when the cramps started. They became so painful that I was terrified that I wouldn't make it to the bathroom in time. I did, but I sat in there crying my eyes out, thinking that I just wanted to be home. It was mortifying to have to ask the guy to take me home. He was real nice about it and even called me for another date, but I knew I could never face him again."

Ann Marie's avoidance of dating led to a very lonely, restricted leisure life. Through therapy, she came to realize that her anxiety about the date and her food choices contributed to the severity of her symptoms. Using anxiety management techniques, careful food planning, and gentle assertion, Ann Marie was able to slowly reintroduce herself to the dating scene. She eventually found a young man who was extremely understanding and supportive of her efforts to cope with her intestinal disorder.

If your mealtimes have become fraught with tension and apprehension, it is time to make some changes in your approach. Remember that meals are designed to replenish the resources—in both our bodies and our souls—that get depleted by the demands of daily life. Taking a few steps to make meals a more pleasant experience is a good idea for everyone, but seems to be essential for a person living with IBS. After all, it might make the difference between feeling good or feeling bad.

Maintain a fairly regular schedule of meals. This will help to regulate your system. Work toward smaller, more frequent meals, as heavy meals tend to stimulate strong, painful intestinal contractions. You should plan for breakfast, lunch, and dinner, plus two or three healthy snacks. Try not to go more than three or four hours without eating something.

Slow down. Create soothing rituals surrounding your meals, whether it be reading the paper with your lunch or always lighting a candle with your dinner. Make the time to eat, so that your body is as relaxed as possible. Don't grab breakfast while you are running out the door. Instead, wake up fifteen minutes earlier. Make time for a sit-down lunch. Set a mood for dinner. Use placemats, have fresh flowers on the table, and turn off the television. If eating with the kids is too hectic, feed them first. Sit with them and discuss their day, then enjoy dinner and conversation with your spouse later on. It doesn't take a lot of effort to pamper yourself, leaving you feeling refreshed, soothed, and satisfied.

Practice Makes Perfect

Although the information in this chapter may seem a bit overwhelming at first, with time and practice, you will find that you are eating in a healthier manner and significantly reducing your intestinal distress by eliminating your personal triggers. Here is a summary of the most important things to remember:

1. Rule out intolerance to lactose and bran.

2. When symptomatic, avoid:
    sugars and artificial sweeteners
    fats
    gas-producing vegetables
    alcohol
    caffeine

3. Slowly increase fiber intake.

4. Drink lots of water.

5. Make mealtimes as regular and relaxing as possible.

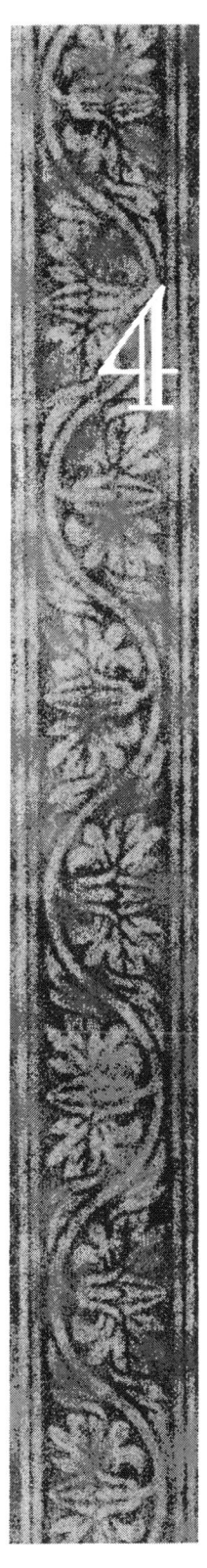

4 Taking Aim at Acute Symptoms

It's time to shoot straight to the heart of the matter. You don't feel well. It stinks to be sick. You know that you need to eat better, start exercising more, and learn how to deal with your stress differently, but for right now you just want to *feel* better. Let's talk about what you can do in the short run to cope with the miserable symptoms of IBS.

Getting a Grip

Your food diary has probably given you a pretty good sense of the predominant symptoms that you're struggling with. I would like you to take a closer look at how those symptoms manifest themselves, not only in terms of how often they rear their ugly heads, and how severe they are, but also how long they last. It would also be helpful at this point to figure out if there's any association between your symptoms and the situations you find yourself in. Like a good spy, the more information you have regarding your enemy, the more power you feel and the greater your chance of victory.

Exercise: Self-Monitoring

This new worksheet resembles your food diary, but instead of recording what you eat, you'll write down the situation that you're in when you experience intestinal distress. Continue to rate your symptoms using a 1 to 5 severity scale. In addition, record next to the symptom how much time elapsed before you began to experience symptom relief.

Self-Monitoring Sheet

Don't forget:
Severity (1 low to 5 high)
Duration (length of symptoms)

Time	Situation	Symptoms

Watch and Learn

To help you visualize how this works, take a look at Walter's self-monitoring sheet:

Walter's Self-Monitoring Sheet

Time	Situation	Symptoms
Mon. 9:45 A.M.	At work—very busy!	Painful cramps - 5 Diarrhea—25 min.
Tues. 10:30 A.M.	Work	Feel constipated - 4 Straining
Wed. all morning	Work	Constipated, unable to go, bloating - 5
Thurs. 10:00 A.M.	Work	Constipated at first, difficult but successful bowel movement - 3
Fri. 8:45 P.M.	Out to dinner	Cramps and diarrhea 10 min. - 4

Walter's job as a news director for a small, local television station is high-paced and demanding. He has little patience for dealing with the intrusiveness of his IBS symptoms. You can see that he appears to alternate between episodes of diarrhea and constipation. He was surprised that his diarrhea episodes were fairly short in duration. "Sometimes, I feel like I'm in the bathroom forever. I am so tense and self-conscious thinking about all the work I should be doing and thinking that everybody must be wondering where the hell I am."

Once he realized that the cramping and diarrhea didn't go on for as long as he imagined, he was better able to relax and let nature take its course. To his surprise, this approach actually resulted in even shorter episodes.

Walter's self-monitoring sheets also gave him useful information regarding the discomfort of constipation. His urges to relieve himself were strongest in the morning. He thus began to make it a point to try to schedule some time each morning to sit on the toilet, relax, read the paper, and hope for the best.

We have only looked at one week of Walter's experience. It would be a good idea for you to keep records over a period of several weeks. If you are still working on your food diary, you can combine the two sheets and gather information on the food that you eat *plus* more specific information regarding the symptoms that you might be experiencing. Follow Walter's example and look for patterns. Are your episodes of cramping and diarrhea really lasting as long as you think they are? Does your system seem to operate under any sort of biological clock? Are certain situations consistently associated with certain symptoms? Take away more of the mystery and you get closer to a solution.

Dealing with Diarrhea

The urgency that generally goes hand in hand with diarrhea has earned it top billing in our discussion of tips for coping with specific IBS symptoms. The distress of diarrhea is further exacerbated by the social shame and embarrassment that is usually inherent in the experience. It can be immensely helpful to remind yourself that diarrhea is a universal experience and therefore one that everyone can empathize with.

Jennifer's story is one that easily elicits sympathy. Jennifer is a sweet, petite high school junior. When Jennifer came to see me, her parents were in the process of separating, and their efforts toward a divorce settlement were marked by an enormous amount of conflict, leaving Jennifer with very torn loyalties. Jennifer described her experience with IBS: "Going to school is such a nightmare! I hate it! I dread it every morning when I wake up. I have to walk to school and as soon as I start to get close, the cramps start. They hurt *so* bad. I have to walk with my butt clenched because I'm so afraid that I'm not going to be able to get to the bathroom on time. I never know if the custodian is going to be there with the keys to let me in. What do I do if he's not there?"

Accidents Rarely Happen

It's easy to understand Jennifer's panic. Most people would find it extremely humiliating to have an accident. Luckily, accidents of this nature, called fecal incontinence, are quite rare in IBS. Your muscle control has been well developed and has certainly received much practice in the years since you were toilet trained.

If you have not yet experienced an accident, you can reassure yourself that it isn't likely to happen. You're probably thinking, because I hear it all the time, "But I just made it in the nick of time." To which I respond, "Precisely." Once you have made it, your body knows that it is okay to relax its hold and, well, you know the rest. If you do struggle with fecal incontinence, we'll discuss some ways of coping with that later on in the chapter.

We have just covered two areas where adjusting your thinking can help to reduce your distress. To review, the first is to remind yourself that other people will be understanding, not judgmental, if they become aware of your diarrhea experience. Instead of thinking, "This is absolutely mortifying," which is a great way to raise your anxiety level and worsen your symptoms, reassure yourself: "Everyone feels like this at one point or another. They know what it's like. If they knew what I was going through they would be kind about it. They aren't going to judge me as a person because of what's happening with my body."

Similarly, instead of thinking "Oh, my God! I'm not going to make it in time!" and sending your anxiety and sense of urgency through the roof, talk to yourself and work to calm yourself down. "Relax, it'll be okay. If I calm down, my body will cooperate and wait until I have found a bathroom before letting loose. It hasn't failed me before and it's not going to fail me now." There's a clear connection between the way that you think and the way that you *feel*.

Time Will Tell

As shown by Walter's example, timing the length of your diarrhea and cramping episodes can be quite helpful. You know that all episodes come to an end. You do eventually get the feeling that everything is out of your system and things are calming down. Having a general sense of how long it takes to get to that point helps you to remember as you are going through it that flare-ups do come to an end. If you remember our discussion about the digestive system, you know that with diarrhea, the muscles are contracting too quickly, moving the material through rapidly. Eventually, there will be no more matter to move along and the contractions will subside. As you are sitting on the throne, it may seem like an eternity. Looking at your watch and reassuring yourself that it will probably be only another ten minutes or so will help to improve your ability to tolerate the rest of the episode. So, sit back, relax, check your watch periodically, and ride it out.

Planning Equals Coping

Another advantage to gathering data regarding the length of your diarrhea distress is that it allows you to plan. (Now there's a concept!) Bernice found this to be a lifesaver. Bernice's self-monitoring sheets revealed that her diarrhea was most likely to flare up just as she was leaving her house to attend a social function. You don't have to be a psychologist to figure out that Bernice obviously has some issues regarding her social confidence. But it's not possible to overcome social anxiety overnight, so Bernice had to make some adjustments. She found it extremely helpful to plan to spend approximately twenty-five minutes in the bathroom before getting into the car. She calmly explained this to her husband, who adjusted his schedule accordingly. When committing to a social engagement, she made sure she left herself with a half hour of leeway regarding the time she would arrive. By covering all her bases, Bernice significantly reduced her self-imposed sense of pressure and her feelings of shame and embarrassment. She and her husband no longer started off each outing with an argument about being late. She finally began to feel that the disorder was no longer ruling her, but that she was once again in charge of her life.

The key word here is planning. Unfortunately, when we are anxious, we are quite susceptible to projecting instead of planning. Projecting involves thinking about the worst-case scenario, without any thought of how one might deal with such. Projections usually sound something like this: "Oh my God! What if that happened? It would be horrible!" What most people forget is that one way or the other, we usually find a way to cope with what is presented to us.

You can prepare yourself for possible contingencies by designing strategies for coping. Consider Bernice's example and think about what you worry about with your diarrhea. Do you experience anticipatory anxiety by worrying about having an episode in certain situations? If so, devise a plan for dealing with it. Your plan may involve adjusting your schedule, asserting your needs to others, or simply visualizing yourself calmly dealing with the situation as it arises. Knowing the average length of your episodes can help significantly with the planning process.

Careful Eating

Be kind to your digestive system. If you've been experiencing diarrhea, treat your body with kid gloves. Now is not the time to be trying out that new Mexican restaurant that just opened up around the corner. Eat plain foods that you know your system can handle. Think about what your mother would give you when you were a little kid and suffered from a stomach virus. Tea (decaf of course), toast (whole wheat of course), ginger ale, and gelatin. If nothing else, the (hopefully) soothing memories of childhood may help you to feel better.

Mom's remedies are consistent with medical recommendations. You may also find that the BRAT diet we discussed in the last chapter is quite helpful. Bananas, rice, applesauce, and toast are all soothing and easy on your system, and they bulk up your stool as well. You will need to slowly increase the fiber in your diet, particularly the soluble kind found in oatmeal, barley, and fruits, particularly apples. Drink plenty of water to help these fiber sources to firm up that watery stool. Drinking water also helps to replace the fluid that is lost during a diarrhea episode.

When experiencing diarrhea, avoid dairy products. Dairy products tend to not be absorbed well during such episodes and thus exacerbate symptoms. This seems to be a temporary state of affairs and does not indicate lactose intolerance. Avoid caffeine, artificial sweeteners, and fatty foods. Even if you're usually okay with these things, you might experience a temporary sensitivity to them during diarrhea flare-ups. Remember, these restrictions don't have to be permanent, but it's prudent to play nice until things calm down.

Should I Tell?

One of the most difficult things about coping with IBS is the shame and secrecy that seem to be inherent in the disorder. True, we live in a society that frowns upon the open discussion of the natural workings of the body, but the effort that it takes to hide your distress from others may be serving to exacerbate that very same distress. For your own sake, consider telling others that you aren't feeling well. Why should it be totally acceptable to leave a party with a bad headache, but not because of the runs? There are ways to keep your modesty but still open the door for support and empathy from others. Don't forget, if roughly 20 percent of the population suffers from IBS, the odds are good that the person you are disclosing to may be a fellow sufferer!

The simplest way to verbalize your discomfort to others is to say, "I'm not feeling well. I'm having trouble with my stomach." Now, that doesn't sound too hard, does it? If you feel that you can't keep saying that over and over again, you can explain that you have a disorder called irritable bowel syndrome. You can describe the syndrome as involving persistent intestinal difficulty and explain that you're working hard to make your life more manageable in spite of the illness. This type of explanation makes it very likely that you will receive understanding and support from those around you. You may even get some helpful tips—and most likely some unwanted advice. You can see that limited disclosure protects your privacy, relieves self-induced pressure, and serves to strengthen interpersonal connections. Beats the pants off of shame and self-consciousness, doesn't it?

Coping with Constipation

This could be a one-word section. Fiber. Fiber is your best defense against constipation. As you now know, fiber serves to bulk up and soften the stool, which is essential so that you can push it out without so much trouble. Remember that with constipation, insoluble fiber is more effective. Since insoluble fiber doesn't dissolve in water, water is retained and helps to lubricate the stool's passage through the system. Insoluble fiber can be found in bran, whole wheat products, and vegetables. Your physcian may recommend that you use a bulking product containing psyllium, a natural substance that serves as a laxative. Although you can buy it over the counter, it is best that you consult with your doctor regarding the optimal dosage. Never use over-the-counter laxatives without permission from your doctor. Chronic use of nonbulking laxatives can alter the functioning of your colon and exacerbate your condition.

Make it a point to drink plenty of water, which helps to lubricate the stool. In addition, if you keep your body well hydrated, your colon will not have to absorb as much water from the stool. If the colon draws too much water from the stool, the stool will become hard and dry, making it very difficult to eliminate.

Regularity

There is one other key word to keep in mind when coping with constipation: regularity. This is a popular conversational topic among a certain age segment of the population. You want to make regularity—in your meals and bowel movements—a life goal. This doesn't mean that you should worry if you don't have a bowel movement every day at the same time. Those old commercials seemed to imply that if your bowels were regular, then the rest of your life would all fall into place. We won't go that far, but you want to start to train your body to empty itself in a predictable way, so it's important to eat on a regular schedule and to make time for regular trips to the bathroom.

Take a look at your self-monitoring sheets. Do you eat your meals at a regular time each day? Is there any sort of pattern to your bowel movements? Does the size of your meals have any relation to the timing of those trips to the bathroom? Eating your meals on some sort of consistent schedule helps your intestinal system begin to operate on its own consistent schedule. Like a well-run train line, you want the food moving along consistently and efficiently until it reaches the end of the line.

Your self-monitoring sheets should help you to determine when your body appears to be more likely to experience a bowel movement. Use this information in your meal planning. Eating a large meal serves to stimulate the gastro-colic reflex, a series of intestinal contractions that push the stool along and prompt the urge to empty your bowels. Once you have pinpointed your most likely time to feel the urge for a bowel movement, you can try to stimulate the reflex by planning a meal around that time. If you are more likely to have a bowel movement in the morning, make sure you take the time to eat a large breakfast. Similarly, if your more probable time is the evening, save your heaviest meal for the end of the day.

In addition to eating your meals at a predictable time each day, you should schedule a regular time to visit the bathroom. Using the information that you have gathered about the optimal time for a movement, have a meal or a hot drink to stimulate the reflex, and then go relax and sit on the john. Men tend to be quite good at this. They often go so far as to say that it's the only time of day when they get any peace. They'll take some sort of reading material and disappear for a while. If you don't already do this, it's time to start.

Deborah swears by this type of scheduling, called bowel retraining. "I used to spend the entire day feeling like I had to go to the bathroom. Half the time I would get there and nothing would happen. Other times I would push and push and only the tiniest little pebble would pop out. I was forced to take a good look at my schedule. I would get the kids off to school and then run around like a maniac trying to get everything done before they came home again. Now I have completely slowed my mornings down. After the kids get on the bus, I sit down and have a big bowl of cereal and read the paper. Then I take the time to use the bathroom and have found that I am usually successful. Taking the time to take care of me first has made a world of difference."

The last tip for coping with constipation is to exercise on a regular basis. In addition to all of the various health benefits of exercise, vigorous exercise can stimulate a bowel movement. (Ask any runner!) It is also a good idea to engage in exercises that strengthen the abdominal muscles. Strong abdominal muscles will help you in your efforts to push out a stool, thus reducing the strain on your anus.

Fecal Incontinence

The name itself is enough to raise anxiety. As stated above, fecal incontinence refers to what most of us would call "having an accident," where fecal matter slips out in a situation other than sitting on a toilet. Luckily, fecal incontinence is fairly rare in IBS, although it has been my experience that most IBS patients are quite worried about its occurrence. With work, you can cope with everything in life, even this.

The best things you can do to cope with fecal incontinence are to be prepared and to work to reduce your feelings of shame and embarrassment. Women deal with the emission of fluids on a monthly basis. Although most women like to keep the matter private, they learn to deal with it in a matter-of-fact way. They make sure that they have access to sanitary products as needed, and they attribute the process to nature rather than to some inner personal failing. Work toward the same attitude for your distressing bowel symptom, and you'll find that your anxiety will lessen significantly.

The same food recommendations for diarrhea hold true for incontinence. If you can reduce the frequency of diarrhea, you will reduce your probability of soiling. Similarly, if you can bulk up your stool with fiber, it is less likely that there will be loose matter to leak out.

The strategies for working toward bowel regularity that we discussed for constipation may also be helpful. If you can stimulate your gastro-colic reflex early in the day by eating a large, fiber-rich breakfast, you may be able to empty your bowels and therefore reduce the chances of having a problem later in the day.

Bloating

One of the major complaints of patients with IBS is the discomfort of bloating. It makes getting dressed a complicated affair. What to wear? "That slinky black dress is out." "Better make sure that there are some extra notches on that belt." "I feel like I'm five months pregnant." The pleasure from wearing clothes that you feel good in seems to be gone.

This is a good time to stop and acknowledge that you have a physical disorder that needs to be dealt with as such. While "acceptance" implies that you have eagerly embraced whatever hardship you think you need to accept, the word "acknowledge" can be so much more helpful. Acknowledge that you have an illness, and make adjustments for it. Acknowledge its existence and the reality of it—but you don't have to like it.

If you experience abdominal bloating on a regular basis, make your decisions accordingly. Buy clothes that look good, but are comfortable. Don't buy tight-fitting, figure-enhancing clothes if you aren't going to be able to wear them. All you'll do is drive yourself crazy trying them on and then rejecting them. Close-fitting clothes may also aggravate your symptoms by serving to trap gas and cause pain. A comfortable, relaxed, happy you is going to appear much more attractive to others than a miserable fashion plate.

Reducing bloating is another good reason to increase your physical activity level. Sitting for long periods of time, whether at work or simply because you are a couch potato, may contribute to bloating. Regular exercise also helps to reduce constipation, which can add to bloating. Last, but by no means least, exercise will tone up your body, helping you to feel proud about the way that you look, instead of self-conscious.

Gas

Here's another potential area for shame and embarrassment. Our culture is far from accepting the regular noises and odors that result from the normal process of digestion. The only exception to this rule is probably a frat house, where social status and flatulence sometimes go hand in hand. For the rest of society, difficulty with excess gas can be quite distressing.

Interestingly enough, IBS sufferers do not seem to experience more gas than other people. The difference seems to be that the gas is experienced as more painful, possibly due to the abnormal visceral sensitivity that we discussed previously. It is also possible that the amount of gas is perceived as excessive just due to the amount of attention that is now given to the whole digestive process, because it has gone so haywire.

Herein lies your first area of intervention. Try to distract yourself when you begin to perceive that you are feeling gassy. If you need to move your bowels, do so, because it may open up the gate to release the trapped gas. If not, just start to think about something else, something significantly more pleasant than the fact that your colon bacteria have set upon something that you ate, causing certain gases to be released by the ensuing chemical reaction!

Don't awfulize. Talk to yourself in a calming manner. "There is nothing to be ashamed of. Everyone's stomach makes funny noises at times. Everyone has experienced having an unpleasant smell come out uninvited. Since they have all been there at one time or another, no one is going to judge me harshly. People will understand."

In order to reduce intestinal gas, you may want to avoid engaging in behaviors that cause you to swallow air, such as smoking, chewing gum, eating too quickly, and talking while eating. In addition, take a look at your food, and choose carefully, depending on the situations that you are likely to be in. Watch out for those gas-producing vegetables, such as broccoli, brussels sprouts, beans, cabbage, peppers, and onions. Avoid drinking carbonated beverages, as they can increase intestinal gas. Spicy food can result in unpleasant odors as well. Don't feel the need to cut these foods out of your diet altogether—just avoid them when you are going to be in a social situation where you don't want to have to deal with gas symptoms. If you are going to be home, have a party!

Nurse Yourself Back to Health

As you can see, the best way to deal with your symptoms is to acknowledge that you are suffering from a real physical disorder and to treat yourself accordingly. Cut yourself some slack and adjust your expectations for yourself. Talk to yourself in a calm, soothing manner, reminding yourself that your physical symptoms are in no way a reflection of who you are as a person and that others will certainly understand if your distress is made known to them (either purposely or inadvertently).

As with many illnesses, changes need to be made as to how you conduct your life. You don't need to be happy about them, but you can be happy with the resulting relief and the reward of regaining control over your life. Eat well, exercise your body, regulate your schedule, and dress comfortably. None of this is painful or distressing. IBS is. It may take some effort at first, but eventually these changes will become routine. You'll find that you not only feel better physically, but that your overall sense of well-being is on the rise.

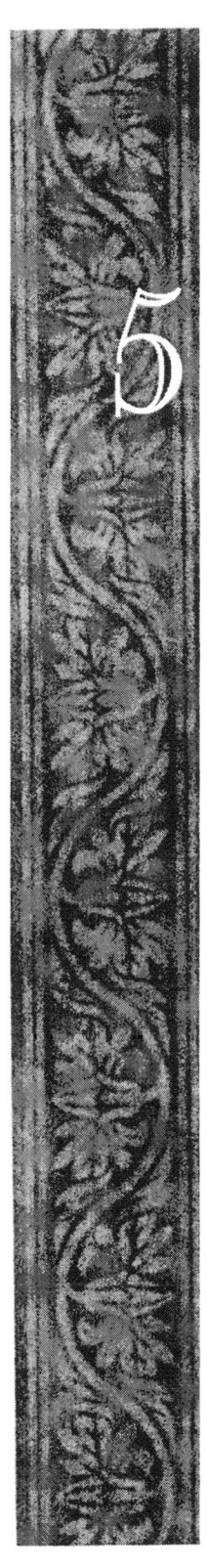

5 Dealing with Difficult Situations

Some people like to use the term "control freak" when describing others, but the truth is that everyone likes to feel a sense of control. We like to feel that we're the masters of our destiny because it reduces our anxiety. A sense of control gives us the illusion that things will be okay, that we can ward off catastrophes. Irritable bowel syndrome wreaks havoc with your sense of control. You never know when it will strike or how bad it will get. It becomes almost impossible to make plans or commit yourself to anything. A simple party invitation fills you with dread rather than excitement. How can you agree to cook a holiday meal if you don't know if you'll be sick as a dog? You can't enjoy planning a vacation because you're worried about having access to a bathroom while you're traveling. The seemingly simple things in life become excruciatingly complicated.

Taking Control

It's time to regain your sense of control and to stop feeling ruled by the unpredictability of your illness. We'll take a look at various situations that are difficult to cope with when you have IBS and discuss strategies for successful management. We'll also work to identify situations that, for one reason or another, trigger your IBS symptoms.

Which Symptoms Affect You?

You have already been gathering this information with your self-monitoring sheets. Now we're going to shift our focus away from the Symptoms column and take a look at the situations in which you're likely to experience distress. Look at your sheets to see if there are any patterns. Are there any situations with which you find it extremely difficult to cope because of your IBS? Are there any particular situations in which your symptoms keep popping up? Identifying the situations that give you difficulty, either because of the interference of IBS or because the situations trigger IBS symptoms, is a good start toward improved management of your illness and easier living.

Although it is generally fairly easy to identify the situations in which IBS is disruptive, situations that serve to trigger IBS symptoms aren't always so obvious. That's why your self-monitoring sheets are so helpful. I worked with a young woman named Caroline whose IBS became overwhelming to her following the birth of her first child. She found coping with her IBS to be so distressing that she completely limited her life. She avoided doing anything that wasn't an absolute necessity. Left to her own devices, she would have stayed home all the time. However, her husband was a very active guy who encouraged her to continue to do the things they did before the baby was born, such as going antiquing, going out to dinner, and visiting friends. Caroline's self-monitoring sheets revealed an interesting pattern. Her episodes of diarrhea were most severe prior to an outing with her husband, but were milder or nonexistent if she planned to take the baby out by herself. This was extremely surprising to me as I would have assumed that Caroline would have felt less anxious when she had her husband around to help her take care of the baby. When I asked her why this might be so, her answer was quite revealing. "Maybe the reason I feel sicker when I go out with my husband is that I'm worried that the baby is going to interfere with his having a good time. You see, he didn't really want to have children. I was the one who pressured him into starting a family."

Caroline was clearly putting herself under tremendous pressure. She felt responsible for how the baby acted on family outings, but anyone who has ever spent five minutes around an infant knows that their behavior is completely unpredictable. Once we had identified the source of Caroline's anxiety, we were able to address it directly. The first thing Caroline did was to objectively try to characterize her husband's feelings about the baby. As she took the time to really think about it, she realized that her husband was crazy about the baby and probably had no regrets about having her. The next thing Caroline did was to actually check this out with her husband, who expressed gratitude to Caroline for talking him into starting a family. Caroline then discussed her fears about the baby disrupting their routines, to which her husband replied that he understood that this was par for the course. For future outings, Caroline was able to ask and rely on her husband to help her out with the baby. Her anxiety decreased dramatically, as did the disruptiveness of her IBS symptoms.

Anticipation

Once you identify situational triggers, you can then develop strategies for reducing your distress. Be on the lookout for *avoided* situations. The mere anticipation of these situations can result in intestinal symptoms. Make sure that you record the anticipatory anxiety as well as the avoided situation on your self-monitoring sheets under the Situation column. This will give you valuable information as to where you need to intervene to return to an active, unrestricted life.

Finding Common Ground

There are certain settings that most IBS patients have difficulty dealing with. We will take a look at some of these hornet's nests, to help you to develop ways of coping with them without getting stung. You may find that you, because of your own individual circumstances, have some troubling situations that aren't covered specifically in this chapter. However, there *are* common elements that make situations challenging for people with IBS, so you will find that the strategies suggested are fairly universal in their application.

Work

Nothing compares to the workplace for a lack of freedom and a lack of privacy. This can make going to work especially difficult for a person with irritable bowel syndrome. The lack of freedom and privacy certainly contribute to the fact that IBS is a major reason for employee absenteeism. It is going to take patience, courage, and creative thinking to learn to balance your self-care needs with your work responsibilities.

Kerry's waitressing job provided no time to be sick, because the restaurant where she worked had a thriving, hectic lunch business. When Kerry first started to experience attacks of pain, cramping, and diarrhea while waiting tables, she thought she was going to be fired. "I kept asking another waitress to cover for me, but she was usually pretty swamped. My manager kept looking for me, wondering where I was. I was afraid she was going to think that I kept runnning to the bathroom to do drugs. I really liked my job and I didn't want to have to give it up, but I didn't know how long I could keep going on like this."

Kerry decided to attack her IBS on two fronts. She began to get up earlier in the mornings to prepare herself a big breakfast, instead of the usual cup of coffee grabbed on the run before her shift started. Although she still had attacks of diarrhea, they usually occurred in the morning before she got to the restaurant, and her system generally stayed pretty quiet for the rest of the day. The other thing that Kerry did was to explain her health status to her manager. She described IBS and talked about what she was doing to try to manage the condition so that it wouldn't affect her work. The manager was very supportive and even offered to cover for Kerry when Kerry needed help.

Should You Tell?

Kerry's experience raises an important question. Should you tell or keep your IBS hidden? From a mental health point of view, disclosure is usually a good thing, but when it comes to people's livelihood, things are not quite that simple. Kerry was lucky—her manager made accommodations for her condition. But unfortunately, not everyone will have such a positive experience.

From a business point of view, telling can be quite risky. Many jobs entail a high degree of competition and any weakness is seen as something to be exploited. Often, if a person is viewed as having an illness that will interfere with performance, they get passed up for certain projects or promotions. Although discrimination due to physical disability is against the law, it doesn't mean that it doesn't happen. Only you can decide whether, in the climate of your particular workplace, telling might ease up your life or make things more difficult.

If you feel safe in disclosing, your assertiveness will really help to decrease the pressure that comes from trying to hide your condition from others. Disclosure reduces shame and secrecy, and it opens the door for support from others. It will help you to better plan your work responsibilities, taking into account the demands and unpredictability of your illness. Disclosure will also work to reduce the amount of sick time that you use, since the workplace will become more amenable to symptom management.

Issues of Trust

In order to make the decision regarding disclosure, you need to consider several factors. The most obvious question is whom to tell. Colleagues are generally less risky, as they are in the same boat and do not have decision-making power regarding your employment status. Helpful colleagues can be called upon to temporarily cover for you when you are feeling ill. In other cases, competition is so fierce among same-line workers that they would be the last people that you would want to tell. Similarly, you need to take stock of the gossip potential among co-workers and ascertain each individual's capacity for confidentiality before telling them about such a private matter.

If you decide that it's safe to tell your boss or supervisor about your IBS and they respond in a supportive manner, you will experience tremendous relief. Think about the pressure that will be removed if you don't have to constantly be worried about covering for yourself and hiding your distress. If you don't feel that your supervisor will be supportive, sometimes enlisting the help of personnel or the human resources department can be useful.

What to Say

I am a firm believer in education. If I weren't I wouldn't have written this book. Ignorance leads to bad judgment and prejudice against others who are viewed as different. Knowledge allows people to be understanding of the distress of others without being judgmental. You'll be doing yourself and others who have IBS a real service if you educate people about the nature of IBS and what it entails. You can tell people that you've been diagnosed with an intestinal illness that results in episodes of pain and difficulty going to the bathroom, and that the illness affects up to 20 percent of the population. You can tell them that the illness is not caused by stress, but that stress makes it worse. You can tell them that you are trying to cope with your illness by being more careful about what you eat and by trying to deal with the stress in your life in some healthier ways. You can then discuss ways in which your job structure can be changed in order to help you to better manage your illness.

Creative Ways of Working

It's possible to make changes in the way things are run at work so as to take into account that your body isn't at its physical best. Compare your typical weekly work schedule to your self-monitoring sheets. Can work responsibilities be scheduled differently so as to be kinder to your system? If you know that you need extra time in the bathroom in the mornings due to constipation, schedule conferences in the afternoon. If you tend to be in the most distress after lunch, try to pencil in that time to complete paperwork so that you aren't beholden to someone else's schedule. This is clearly where creative thinking comes in.

Look at your self-monitoring sheets to see if there is any relationship between particular job activities and your IBS symptoms. Once you have identified any triggers, you can actively problem-solve different ways of handling them so as to reduce your anxiety and physical discomfort. Some ideas for dealing with common areas of difficulty are discussed below.

Deadline Dread

Some people are highly reactive to deadlines. The thought of not meeting the deadline can be quite anxiety-provoking and can set off a sensitive intestinal system. When you're faced with a deadline, spend five minutes outlining a *realistic* plan for completing the assignment on time. When planning, don't forget to factor in time spent dealing with your body. Remind yourself to be calm, and tell yourself that you'll complete the work on time. Take a realistic view of what the consequences would really be if some unforeseen event prevented you from meeting the deadline. Very rarely are there catastrophic effects. The bottom line is that the calmer you are in facing the deadline, the more efficiently you will use your time and the more cooperative your body will be.

Public Speaking Paranoia

Public speaking tends to be another universal anxiety-provoker, and one that causes particular dread for the average IBS sufferer. "What if I need to run to the bathroom in the middle of my presentation?" You know what? It wouldn't be the end of the world. Most audiences love a short break to stretch their legs and clear their heads. However, as you would probably prefer that this not happen, there are certainly things that you can do to reduce the risk of a symptom flare-up. The first is to normalize the nervousness that comes with speaking before an audience. A little bit of anxiety is actually helpful in that it motivates you to be prepared and sharpens your senses. If you know that you're scheduled to give a presentation, be careful about what you eat for a day or two ahead of time. Make sure you allow yourself plenty of time to use the bathroom prior to the scheduled start of the talk. Use deep breathing and muscle relaxation techniques (discussed later in this book) to keep your baseline anxiety low. Visualize yourself handling the situation calmly if you do have a problem. That way you won't panic if you start to feel your system acting up. You can excuse yourself, suggest that the audience take a break or review what you have already gone over, and then take the time to tend to your needs. Again, you naturally don't want to have to deal with an IBS flare-up, but you certainly can survive one.

Conference Conundrums

Conferences are similar to public speaking because of the sense of public scrutiny that is involved. Don't be in denial of your physical condition and just hope for the best. Careful planning and not allowing yourself to awfulize the situation can help you cope. When possible, try to schedule meetings and conferences at your most IBS-friendly times. Eat carefully and thoughtfully prior to the meeting. Use relaxation techniques to keep yourself as calm as possible. If you need to use the bathroom, excuse yourself. It's not like this is that unusual a request! Although not everyone suffers from IBS, the need to use a bathroom *is* a universal experience.

Parties

Super Bowl. A crowded party. A nightmare for Tina. "I was sitting there enjoying the game, when all of a sudden I started to experience severe gas pains. At first, I tried to ignore them, hoping they would go away. No luck. They just kept coming and coming until finally I excused myself and went into the bathroom. Unfortunately, the house I was at had only one bathroom and it was right off of the living room where everyone was watching the game. I felt like I was in there forever, and that everyone was wondering what I was doing in there. To make matters worse, a little kid started banging on the door saying that he needed to go the bathroom. I was mortified."

Does this scenario sound familiar to you? Social gatherings, including parties, are rife with two of the major triggers for IBS symptoms: anxiety and food. Without preparation, they can be a disaster waiting to happen. Some people with IBS avoid parties altogether, because they are just too stressful. This is a shame. Parties are meant to be times of enjoyment, a break from your ordinary routine. They provide an opportunity to connect with others, have a few laughs, and enjoy eating interesting food that you don't have to prepare yourself. Getting yourself back into the party circuit is good for you. Doing it is a two-step process.

Step 1: Plan Ahead to Enjoy Yourself

The first step involves learning to manage your IBS and still enjoy yourself when in the company of others. A little perspective always helps. People with more severe bowel disease are in some cases given a colostomy, which involves the use of a pouch worn outside the body that does the job of a colon. Sometimes they have to deal with leakage or odors. They still go to parties. The point here is that you have the right to live your life, even though your colon is giving you trouble. Those around you aren't going to make as big a deal of your difficulties as you think they will.

Careful preparation is key. Be careful with what you eat prior to the party, so as to minimize any adverse reactions. Have a plan drawn up as to how you would handle things if you were to run into a problem. What would you say to people? Where could you find access to a bathroom? What would you say if you really felt the need to leave? Practice how you would explain yourself to others ahead of time. This will reduce your panic if you have difficulty on the spot. Before the party, use relaxation techniques and calming self-talk to keep anticipatory anxiety to a minimum. Remind yourself that even if you get sick, you will manage.

At the party, eat carefully. Eat lightly and avoid those really fatty goodies that always seem to be abundant at parties. Minimize your alcohol intake. You'll be kinder to your stomach and you will be more in control if you have to deal with any sort of physical distress. If you need to use the bathroom, excuse yourself. If you need to leave, just say so. It's nothing to be embarrassed about.

If you make it to a party, you've been successful. If you're able to enjoy yourself for some of the time, even better. If you can stick it through to the end, congratulations! You have defeated the demon.

Step 2: Let Go of Party Anxiety

The second step involves learning to reduce anxiety, not about IBS, but anxiety related to going to parties. Again, parties are meant to be fun! As you know, many things in life are stressful. But, parties shouldn't be. Some people thrive in a party atmosphere. If that's you, you can skip this section. For everyone else, a change in attitude and approach can reduce pre-party jitters and increase party pleasure.

Many people experience anxiety before a party because they don't have confidence in their conversational skills. All you really need to be a good conversationalist is to be a good listener. People love to talk about themselves! Ask them about their life, listen to their response, ask a follow-up question, and you have a lively conversation going. Too often, people focus on their own insecurity, e.g. "I'm not funny enough" or "I'm boring." This internal focus interferes with your ability to enjoy talking with another person. Keep the focus off yourself and on the person you're speaking with, and you'll be just fine.

In addition to asking others to talk about their lives, think about what you have in common and talk about that. This is the reason for so much heated discussion about weather, as it is the one thing that everyone has in common. At a party, you generally have the host and hostess as a mutual acquaintance, and this can be a good jumping-off place for a conversation.

You can also talk about local happenings, current events, and popular movies and books, again all reflecting common areas of interest.

Remember that it takes two to tango, and two to have a conversation. If, despite your efforts, the conversation dries up, move on (you can always go to the bathroom, ha ha). Don't berate yourself. If the other person doesn't hold up their end of the conversation, this is not your fault, and it's not a reflection of your self-worth either. Believe it or not, the other person may simply lack social skills. Also, don't feel that you have to be the life of the party to be well regarded by others. If everyone was loud and needed to be the center of attention, a party would quickly turn obnoxious. A good party needs some Ed McMahon types, the people who laugh at the jokesters. So sit back, enjoy finding out about the lives of others, listen to the jokes, and have fun.

Holidays

Holidays are a lot like parties, but you can now add a third trigger to the IBS mix: family members. Despite what you might have seen on television, most family gatherings are not as stress-free as those of the Walton and Brady households. For those of us who are living in the real world, holidays can be a significant source of stress and thus may significantly affect IBS symptoms.

Sarah, a thirty-two-year-old mother of two, was not surprised when her self-monitoring sheets showed a pattern of symptom outbreaks that coincided with holiday celebrations with her parents and siblings. "Family get-togethers are excruciating. The tension level is so high. It doesn't take much for a shouting match to break out. When I'm there, my stomach is a quivering bunch of nerves. I realized that I usually get sick right after I get home from one of these visits. I'm beginning to think that my family is hazardous to my health!"

Family Drama

As you can see, holidays spent with family members can be a potential hot spot for people with IBS. Whether it be dealing with an overbearing, intrusive relative, feeling trapped into playing a role set down in childhood, or dealing with outright conflict, family dynamics can be challenging. Combine that with food that is generally overabundant and fatty, and alcohol that is often too prevalent, and you have a recipe for disaster. Identifying your particular triggers can help you to pinpoint areas for intervention.

As with other difficult situations, watch what you eat and work to keep your anxiety level as low as possible. Look for the factors that make a holiday extra stressful for you and brainstorm ways to reduce that stress. Do you take on too much responsibility for meal planning or party setup? If so, delegate. Don't feel that you have to do it all. Are you too much of a perfectionist, so that you drive yourself crazy making sure that everything is just right? Let it go. It's okay if things are just good enough. Remember, you have a right to make accommodations for yourself, because it isn't healthy to be doing something for others that is harmful to you, IBS or not.

Role Playing

Some people feel locked into playing a certain role with members of their family. Often these roles are set down in childhood. This feeling of being expected to behave in a certain way can trigger feelings of resentment and anxiety. Examine the role that you play in your family. Are you the entertainer, the peacemaker, the do-it-all, or the attention-craver? Take the time to ask yourself if you want to remain locked into that role rather than being free to just be yourself. Does it do you any harm to continue the same pattern of behavior? Does it exacerbate your IBS? Think about making some changes. Are you afraid? If so, why? Are you afraid of how others might react? How could you handle this if they do? Freeing yourself up to be yourself is good self-care. If it helps you to feel better, both physically and emotionally, how can that be a bad thing? Remember that if you are feeling better, you have more to offer other people. You are thus doing yourself and your family a good service.

Conflict

Families are often hotbeds for conflict. The closeness of the bond, ongoing sibling rivalries, and parent–adult child struggles regarding boundaries and independence all serve to increase the potential for trouble. Your job is to strike a balance between setting limits on others regarding your rights and feelings and acting as an ambassador to keep the peace. Beware of leaning too far to one side or the other. Keep calm, keep a sense of humor, and remember that you don't have to like the members of your family—you just have to get along with them for the duration of the holiday visit.

Understanding and Support

Lest we cast such a gloomy view of families, let us say that in some cases, family members can be a valuable resource in coping with a chronic condition like IBS. Because of the familiarity and security that is inherent in most families, you can perhaps feel freer about discussing your struggles with IBS. This can provide an opportunity to avail yourself of priceless support. You need not be so worried about negative judgments of you by others, because no one knows you as well as your family and their view of you is probably already quite well established. Holidays can provide a time to share recollections of previous happy times, help to connect you to your roots, and remind you of the safety net that family provides. Avoiding holidays because of your IBS will prevent you from enjoying these positive benefits. Careful planning, healthy eating, and the use of good interpersonal skills can help you to manage your IBS and your clan.

Restaurants

Going out to eat is supposed to be a treat. For one thing, you don't have to cook or clean up! You get to choose from a variety of foods, eat in a relaxed, comfortable setting, and experience the conversation and attention of others. IBS, once again, can interfere with the enjoyment of one of life's pleasures. There are several potential pitfalls common to IBS sufferers that lead them to avoid dining out. The goal is to avoid the pitfalls, not the restaurants.

If dining out is an important part of your life due to social or business demands, it is well worth the effort to develop new techniques that will decrease your physical and emotional distress. Some people avoid restaurants altogether, but avoidance is never a good solution to a problem. Avoidance gets rewarded due to a short-term decrease in anxiety, but then results in increased anxiety whenever the avoided situation is considered. Exposure, or facing the object of your fear, is the best way to reduce anxiety. As you walk through the scary situation, you learn strategies for managing the situation and thus reduce the fear. Think about it this way: Even if you can arrange your life so that you never eat in a restaurant, you are depriving yourself of a pleasurable experience, preventing yourself from overcoming your anxiety, and allowing your IBS to unnecessarily restrict your life.

Recipe for Disaster

The major mistake that many people with IBS make is to try to eat very lightly or even skip a meal or two in anticipation of dining in a restaurant. Then, when they get there, they eat a large, heavy meal, perhaps made up of many courses. This eating schedule can play havoc with your system. Remember that eating a heavy meal stimulates the gastro-colic reflex, which stimulates colon contractions. The heavier the meal, the stronger the contractions. For a person with IBS, strong contractions can translate into painful cramps and diarrhea. It is much better to eat your meals on a consistent schedule to encourage your system to consistently process the food. If you are going to avoid anything, avoid eating too large an amount of food while dining out. Again, this doesn't mean deprivation—just save some of the typically large portions for the next day. (Hey, you get two meals for the price of one.)

Eating in a restaurant also puts people at risk for unhealthy food choices. Too much alcohol can set off a skittish system. Rich, creamy, and deep-fried foods, all typical restaurant fare, are usually associated with a high fat content. As you know, fatty foods contain the hormone CCK, which is also known to stimulate intestinal contractions. Making wise food choices is essential to surviving and enjoying a restaurant meal.

Escape Hatches

Another potential area of difficulty for IBS patients considering a meal in a restaurant has to do with the feeling of being trapped. Regina describes this well: "I'm usually apprehensive before I even get to the restaurant, wondering if I'm going to get sick. As soon as the waiter or waitress takes the order, I panic. Now I am committed. What if I get sick? What if I just need to go home? Once I order the food, I feel so trapped. I know I can't just get up and leave." This anxiety spike was so uncomfortable for Regina that she began to refuse to go out to eat.

Regina's anxiety was based on faulty thinking. There are very few situations in adulthood where a person is truly trapped. Ordering a meal in a restaurant is certainly not one of them. Placing an order only obligates you to pay for the food, not necessarily to stay and eat it. Once Regina began to think more rationally about the subject, she was able to envision a plan in which she left money on the table and left the restaurant if she thought that was what she needed to do. With this escape hatch in mind,

Regina was able to significantly reduce her anxiety, calm down her body, and begin to once again frequent her favorite eateries.

Travel

The same entrapment fear is prominent in many IBS patients' avoidance of travel. The most common fear is of being stuck in some form of transportation with no access to a bathroom. Again, this fear is based on an irrational thought. As I have said before, although not everyone suffers from IBS, everyone has a frequent need to use a bathroom. Therefore, public rest rooms are usually in great supply.

Make Allowances

Acknowledging that you have a greater need for access to the bathroom than the average person can help you to devise travel plans with which you feel comfortable. People with physical disabilities are able to travel, and so can you. Their travel itinerary reflects their need for accessible facilities. Similarly, your itinerary should reflect your need to know that you can get to a bathroom should you need one. Planning out your trip with this in mind can help you to see that traveling with IBS is definitely possible. This kind of planning, as opposed to anxious projection, can help you to keep yourself calm, thus maximizing the chances that your system will also remain calm.

Many forms of public transportation—including airplanes, trains, and even some buses—have rest rooms available. If the rest room is in use, keep calm. The odds are in your favor that your body will wait. If traveling by car or taxi, remember that there are plenty of places where you can pull over to relieve yourself. Social embarrassment or modesty should never keep a person from accessing a bathroom for their own personal comfort.

Illusions of Safety

The other type of faulty thinking that people with IBS are prone to, and which results in making the thought of traveling quite anxiety-provoking, is the illusion that one is safer (e.g. less likely to get sick) in one's own home. Richard is an individual whose belief in this illusion of safety significantly stalled his progress up the career ladder. After his IBS manifested itself, Richard refused to go on any more business trips.

Richard's medical history showed that he had suffered a very severe intestinal virus while on a business trip several years earlier. When this occurred, he was quite ill, running a very high fever, and experiencing vomiting and diarrhea. He was terribly frightened and felt very alone, and the experience really shook him up. Following that illness, he began to experience recurrent episodes of painful cramping and diarrhea and was given the diagnosis of irritable bowel syndrome. Due to his fear of a reoccurrence, he refused to go on any more business trips.

What Richard neglected to realize was that IBS is not triggered by being away from home. IBS is exacerbated by many factors, not all of them known, but attacks can happen anywhere. If you experience symptoms while away from home, these symptoms are most likely triggered by anxiety, not geography. While it may be true that you feel more comfortable in your own home, staying home all the time can lead to a very narrow existence. The benefits of leaving home, opening yourself to new opportunities and new relationships, certainly outweigh the slight advantage of being in your own home if you're going to be sick. In other words, if being sick is pretty much inevitable, maybe it is better to be stuck in a bathroom in a place like Rome, rather than the bathroom in your own house. At least when you start feeling better, the views will be much more interesting.

In Richard's case, we examined the factors of his travel experience that were so traumatic to him. Running a high fever and not knowing what was wrong contributed to Richard's terror, but he could have had the same experience in his own home. Although he was away from home, he was still able to access medical care. It was just bad luck that he got sick while out on the road and the odds of it happening again were quite slim. He might experience intestinal distress due to his IBS, but he will not run a fever, leading to feelings of vulnerability and fears of dying. He reminds himself that IBS is not life-threatening, and that managing symptoms of IBS in a strange hotel room is really no different than managing them at home. Thinking along these lines has helped Richard to again commit to business travel, which has opened the door for salary increases and promotions.

Cross-Situational Strategies

As you can see, many of the strategies discussed for specific situations are really applicable to a variety of situations. It is important to acknowledge your illness without giving in to it. Careful planning is essential. Work out a sensible food plan to minimize food triggers for IBS symptoms. Plan out access routes to bathrooms. Keep your baseline anxiety low by using relaxation techniques. Don't fall into the avoidance trap. Face the feared situation armed with strategies for coping and develop the confidence that comes with success. Opening yourself up to all the experiences that come with exposing yourself to a variety of situations will enrich your life and make you a more interesting person, not just a person defined by having IBS.

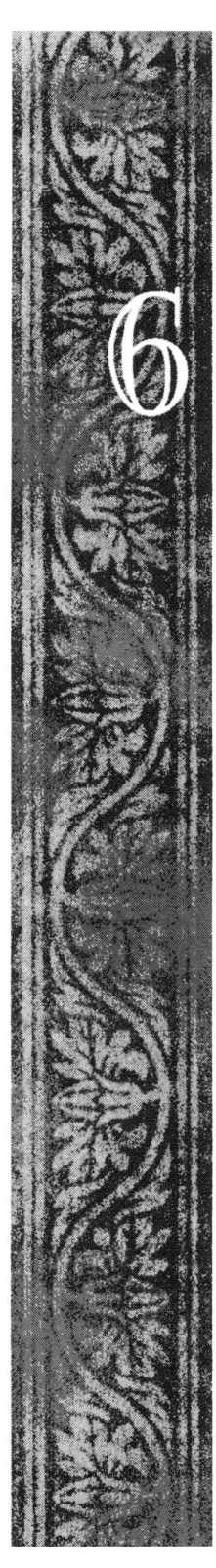

6 Improving Your Emotional Awareness

Gut reaction. Butterflies in the stomach. Bowels in an uproar. Stomach in a knot. These everyday expressions reflect the effect that emotional reactions can have on our body, or more specifically, our digestive system. These effects are magnified when a person has irritable bowel syndrome. For this reason, it's very important to be aware of your emotional reactions and to deal with these in a healthy manner. Whenever possible, you want to avoid inflaming this tender area, and emotional awareness is an invaluable tool.

Getting in Touch

Emotions are the feelings we get in response to outside events or our perceptions of these events. They provide us with extremely important information regarding the circumstances of our life. Is the environment a hostile one, or is it providing us with what we need to fulfill our desires and preferences? This feedback helps us make decisions about how to deal with the world around us.

This concept is extremely important, yet people rarely bring it to the forefront of their consciousness. Emotions play a role in our lives similar to that of physical pain. If you place your hand on a hot surface, you'll feel a painful, burning sensation that will prompt you to remove your hand. A raging toothache signals you to the presence of infection and motivates you to get treatment to resolve the problem. Healthy emotional functioning involves acknowledging your emotional reactions to things and using that information as a cue for coping with our world.

Internal Road Map

When you listen to and validate your emotions, you provide yourself with a great aid for smart decision making. After all, decisions are merely choices, and good decisions are simply those that turn out to have more good consequences than bad ones. No decision is a perfect one, and people often agonize about doing the right thing. When you pay attention to how you feel about each of the options available to you, you get a better sense of which option is more consistent with your desires and preferences. People rarely regret decisions that are consistent with their gut feelings; regret comes along when you say to yourself, "I knew I shouldn't have done that."

Improving your emotional awareness also can lead to active problem solving. Just as feeling a change in the temperature can lead you to change clothes, emotions can lead you to behave in a way that is in your best interest. Feeling angry when you perceive that someone is taking advantage of you can prompt you to assert yourself and protect your own interests. Feeling bored or dissatisfied at work can motivate you to initiate a job search.

It's Personal

Emotional reactions are a highly personal thing. Although there is common ground in terms of how most people will respond to a given environmental event, there is no guarantee that all people will respond in the same way. This means that each of us is responsible for our own emotional reaction. Other people might do things that trigger a reaction in us, but we are the ones who determine what that reaction might be. Similarly, other people are responsible for how they react to our actions. Although we all say things like "He made me so mad," it's technically not true. It is our *interpretation* of the event, based on our own personality and past experiences, that determine our reactions.

For example, let's say that you divulge your IBS troubles to a friend, who responds that this kind of so-called illness is really only a cry for attention. Most of you would be quite angry at this person's insensitivity. On the other hand, you might react with self-doubt, questioning that maybe you really are just imagining everything. Others might respond with anxiety, worrying that they are somehow subconsciously bringing IBS upon themselves. Same trigger, different emotional reaction.

These individual differences also manifest themselves in the way a person's body responds to stress. Some bodies respond with muscle tension, resulting in headaches, whereas others respond with cardiovascular changes, which lead to high blood pressure. Many people respond with gastrointestinal symptoms. The difference with IBS is that these gastrointestinal symptoms are stronger and more chronic.

Stress-Related Illnesses

Although no one knows exactly why stress-related illnesses manifest themselves, scientists have tried to explain the relationship between stress and the development of a physical disorder. As you read this section, think about what factors may have contributed to the development of IBS in your body. Having a better understanding of why this has happened to you can help to reduce unnecessary, unearned, and certainly fruitless self-blame.

Researchers have come up with a working hypothesis regarding stress-related illnesses. The prevailing theory is that individuals respond to stressors in a particular way, activating certain body systems, for example, muscular, cardiovascular, or gastrointestinal. Most of the time, these systems return to a normal state of functioning once the stress has passed. In some cases, however, this return to normalcy does not occur, resulting in chronic symptoms that aren't always directly related to outside factors. There are several possible reasons why this happens. Let's discuss these possibilities as they relate to IBS.

The first possibility is a genetic predisposition toward a breakdown in functioning of one particular system. Popular wisdom certainly supports the notion that IBS runs in families. I've often heard patients say, "My whole family is like this. Whenever we get stressed, we're running to the bathroom."

A second possibility is that of an accident or injury to the system. Studies that have found a relationship between gastroenteritis and the onset of IBS support this explanation. Think about your own experience. Did you have a severe bout of the stomach flu or food poisoning three to six months prior to the onset of your chronic symptoms? It may be that something about that illness left your system overly sensitized.

A third possibility is that the system breaks down due to persistent activation in the face of prolonged stress. In other words, the system burns itself out. The studies showing that an overwhelmingly high number of IBS patients were the victims of physical and sexual abuse in childhood are consistent with this theory. It may be that the abnormally high exposure to such trauma overstimulates the system, eventually leading to chronic malfunction.

Fight-or-Flight Response

When seeking to understand the role of stress in physical illness, it is also helpful to know about the fight-or-flight reflex, which is the body's reaction to a crisis. It is thought to have been developed back when we were living in caves and confronted with all sorts of life-threatening events. If you wandered out of your cave and all of a sudden you were confronted by a hungry-looking lion, you would certainly need the ability to react quickly. In a situation like that, your choices would be to either put up a good fight or run like hell. Thus, the aptly named reflex.

The fight-or-flight response is thought to involve the adrenaline system, with body systems that are needed to deal with the crisis going into high gear. When this response is activated, we experience a heightened awareness of our surroundings, muscle tension, and rapid respiration.

Nonessential systems are relaxed. This accounts for the sensation of a loosening of the bowels when a person is very frightened. This adrenaline reaction is considered to be a deeply ingrained human response to stress.

In today's society, threatening events are not nearly so dramatic, but our exposure to stress has become much more frequent. When our alarm system is activated too often, it appears to be vulnerable to breakdown. As discussed in chapter 1, it has been shown that IBS is often preceded by a significantly stressful event, such as a death or a marital separation. It may be that the prolonged nature of the stress of these events contributes to the development of IBS symptoms.

What Makes a Person Susceptible?

Certain personality factors have also been associated with a vulnerability to stress-related illnesses. This does not in any way imply that you are the *cause* of your distress. Many factors, including your upbringing, your life experiences, and your individual personality, affect how you and your body deal with stress. You might want to spend some time thinking about your parents' response to illness and their attitudes toward your bowel functioning. Have you had any traumatic experiences that have resulted in an overattentiveness to physical symptoms? Do you constantly internalize your emotional reactions, suffering in silence? As you think about your personality and your life, you may gain some insight into reasons for your vulnerability to an illness exacerbated by stress.

The experience of one of my patients provides a dramatic example of this. Joe is a very nice guy whose IBS interfered with his ability to travel by public transportation. Joe was in sales and worked a local territory, so his fears did not cause a problem on an everyday basis. However, they did preclude him from leisure travel. One day, as we discussed whether any childhood events might have predisposed Joe to the development of IBS, Joe grew quite upset. He told me that his parents were both alcoholics who would frequently go out drinking at night, leaving their three children locked in the car. Joe recalled the anguish of being locked in the car with his two sisters and having no access to a bathroom when he needed one. It is certainly possible that these traumatic childhood experiences have contributed to Joe's fear of being trapped in a public place with no access to a bathroom should he need one. These experiences may also be at the root of Joe's hypervigilance toward internal sensations regarding the need to use the bathroom. Joe's anxiety and hypervigilance definitely served to exacerbate his IBS symptoms. Breaking the connection between his childhood experiences and his current fears has helped Joe to reduce his anxiety. He has developed calming self-statements to remind himself that as an adult he has significantly more options and freedom than he did as a child. Planning ahead in terms of guaranteeing himself access to a bathroom enabled Joe to book and enjoy an island vacation.

IBS and Emotional Illness

Although it is well documented that IBS and mood disorders often go hand in hand, the reason is not currently known. Does IBS create anxiety and depressive symptoms or do anxiety and depressive disorders add to the risk of a person developing IBS? A third possibility is that the same factors contribute to the onset of both, resulting in a central physiological malfunction that causes both conditions. In any case, it is essential that you recognize the symptoms of these disorders so that you can avail yourself of appropriate treatment.

Depression

Depression is the most common and most often treated of the mental illnesses, affecting up to 15 percent of the population at some time in their lives. It's different from the down moods that everyone experiences in that it involves a much more prolonged low mood as well as physical symptoms that interfere with normal functioning. Specifically, the symptoms are as follows:

- depressed mood
- crying spells
- difficulty sleeping
- change in appetite/weight
- fatigue; lack of energy and motivation
- difficulty concentrating
- social avoidance
- lack of pleasure from activities
- suicidal thoughts
- feelings of worthlessness, hopelessness, excessive guilt

Significant changes in sleep, appetite, and energy level strongly suggest the presence of a clinical depression. The theory is that the balance of certain brain chemicals called neurotransmitters becomes disrupted, resulting in these diverse symptoms. Suicidal thoughts should always be taken seriously and require *immediate* intervention. Depressed individuals are at extremely high risk for death by suicide.

Generalized Anxiety Disorder

Generalized anxiety disorder (GAD) is manifested by the experience of chronic anxiety, worry, and anticipatory apprehension. The anxiety is sometimes referred to as free floating, because it often does not appear to have a specific trigger. Of all of the anxiety disorders, GAD is the one most frequently diagnosed in patients who have IBS. The symptoms of GAD are:

- excessive worry and anxiety
- feelings of restlessness
- irritability
- muscle tension
- sleep disturbance

Many IBS patients develop severe anticipatory anxiety, which can significantly impair their ability to commit to any type of scheduled social function. At times, the commitment itself is enough to cause a huge anxiety spike. This may be something that happens to you. The fear of experiencing excessive gas or diarrhea, makes it extremely difficult to even think about being out in public.

Panic Disorder

Panic disorder is characterized by episodes of high anxiety, called panic attacks, which seem to occur out of the blue. The symptoms of a panic attack are as follows:

- a feeling of intense anxiety
- heart palpitations
- sweating
- rapid breathing

- trembling
- nausea
- dizziness
- choking sensation
- thoughts that one is dying or going crazy

Panic disorder is seen in approximately two to five percent of the population. For some individuals, the fear of experiencing panic attacks results in agoraphobic avoidance of any situation in which the person perceives that a panic attack might occur. This avoidance can become so severe that the person ends up leading a very restrictive lifestyle. Even without panic disorder, IBS patients often develop a similar kind of avoidance of situations in which they might experience a flare-up of IBS symptoms.

Getting Help

If you see yourself in any of the above descriptions, you may want to make an appointment with a mental health professional to get an accurate diagnosis and to discuss treatment options. If you are experiencing *any* suicidal thoughts, it is absolutely imperative that you be seen by a qualified person immediately. Similarly, if the symptoms of your mood disorder are so severe that they are significantly interfering with your ability to function, mental health treatment is essential.

Where Do I Go?

Many people get easily confused about the difference between a psychiatrist and a psychologist. Although both are trained in the diagnosis and treatment of mental illness, there are some important distinctions. Psychiatrists are trained physicians and thus are able to treat your symptoms through the use of medication. Psychologists receive more in-depth training in the use of psychotherapy, and also perform psychological testing, which can be very useful when the diagnostic picture is not clear. Social workers also conduct psychotherapy and generally have the added advantage of knowing how to access social service resources. Some patients will see a psychologist or social worker for psychotherapy, while their psychiatrist provides medication management. Identifying your particular needs ahead of time can help you to decide which type of professional would best serve you.

Is Medication the Answer?

There is a wide variety of medications available to treat anxiety and depression. Antidepressant medication, in addition to relieving the symptoms of depression, also has an antianxiety effect. A new class of antidepressants, called SSRIs, work to balance the level of serotonin, a neurotransmitter, and have a minimum of unpleasant side effects. You may have heard of some of these medications, such as Prozac, Paxil, and Zoloft. In some cases, antidepressants are prescribed to people with IBS due to their pain-relieving effects.

Benzodiazepines are antianxiety medications, such as Valium and Xanax. These medications work very quickly and effectively at reducing excessive anxiety. However, they can be habit-forming and, when used regularly, can result in an increase in anxiety. If the use of medication is indicated, a good relationship with your doctor is essential in helping you to decide which is the best medication for you.

Psychotherapy has repeatedly been shown to be as effective as medication for the treatment of anxiety and depression. You may be wondering how this is possible if the basis for the mood disorder is chemical. Well, just as stress can have a negative effect on your emotional functioning, managing your stressors more effectively can serve to reverse the malfunction. In addition to having no unpleasant physical side effects, psychotherapy generally produces longer-lasting results. For some individuals, a combination of psychotherapy and medication is the most effective.

Through this book, you are being exposed to many of the principles of a kind of psychotherapy called cognitive behavioral therapy. You may find that personal issues, whether they be a very high current stress level or unresolved issues from childhood, are preventing you from fully benefiting from the strategies presented in this book. If this is the case, a course of psychotherapy may be indicated. A good therapist-patient relationship is crucial for treatment success, so if you don't feel comfortable with the first person you meet, try someone else.

Labeling Your Emotions

Now that we've looked at emotional illness, let's talk about healthy emotional functioning. The first step in learning how to successfully process your emotional reactions is to learn to label them. This may sound simple, but many people don't know how to do it.

Thoughts Aren't Feelings

In general, when people think they are talking about their *feelings*, they are usually describing their *thoughts*. They then become frustrated because other people don't understand them. Mary will say, "I feel that that was so unfair." John will say, "I feel that you were way out of line." These are not feelings, these are points of view. Mary is probably feeling outraged and John is probably feeling angry. Neither one said so, and they will both walk away from the conflict thinking that the other person "just doesn't get it." If people expressed their feelings more directly, and their listeners said "I can see how you would feel that way," conflict would get settled very quickly and the world would be a much better place. But, then again, psychologists would be out of work!

If you want to improve your ability to be in touch with and express your emotions, use feeling words. Remember back in first grade when your teacher would list a variety of emotions on the blackboard? Here are some examples:

happy	frustrated
overjoyed	irritable
excited	angry
relieved	resentful
upset	bitter
disappointed	sad
frightened	sorrowful
anxious	lonely
terrified	grieving

The ability to label your emotions helps you to validate them. I always tell my patients, "If you learn nothing else from me, remember that your emotional reactions are always valid." The thinking on which they are based might be faulty, and your behavioral response might not always be wise, but your feelings are always valid. Your feelings are valid simply because they are yours.

We aren't held accountable for our feelings; we simply have them. We *are* responsible for our behaviors. Remember how Jimmy Carter confessed that he had committed adultery in his mind on many occasions? He had lustful feelings, which aren't a sin, but simply a reaction to external cues. The fact that he remained faithful in his behavior is what's important.

Labeling and validating your emotions will also increase your ability to successfully assert yourself. Assertiveness skills will be covered more fully in chapter 9. For the purpose of this discussion, however, keep in mind that it's difficult for others to understand what you're feeling if you aren't too clear on it yourself!

Healthy versus Unhealthy Emotions

Although all emotions are valid ones, they can be categorized as healthy and unhealthy. Healthy emotions are those that are a direct, natural response to external triggers. For example, fear brought on by confrontation with a snarling dog would be a healthy emotional response. Note that an emotion doesn't have to be a pleasant one to be considered healthy.

Unhealthy emotions usually involve a faulty thought process. As an example, you might experience anxiety due to worrying about having intestinal distress during Thanksgiving Day dinner. This anxiety is a result of the thought "What if I get so sick that I can't sit down and eat with the rest of the family?" This type of thinking is faulty because there is no way to predict the future, and it presupposes that the feared event would be a total catastrophe. The corresponding anxiety is useless because it is causing distress in the present, even though the holiday might be weeks away.

A healthy emotional reaction to the thought of Thanksgiving dinner would be that of concern. If you have a history of experiencing painful intestinal distress during social gatherings that involve a large amount of food, it would be reasonable to be concerned about getting sick. This concern can then prompt you to be prepared, for example by giving careful attention to what you eat and practicing calming self-talk and appropriate assertiveness. This kind of preparation can help make the event a manageable one as opposed to a disaster.

Emotional reactions and thought processes have a close relationship. Methods for identifying and challenging your faulty thinking will be discussed in the next two chapters. In the meantime, keep in mind the following breakdown between healthy and unhealthy emotions when identifying your emotional reactions.

Healthy	Unhealthy
reactive anger frustration resentment	prolonged anger
fear apprehension concern	anxiety
remorse regret	guilt

Feelings Column

It's time for new self-monitoring sheets. As you can see by the form below, from now on I want you to also record any relevant emotions you might have when experiencing IBS symptoms. This column should only contain emotion words. Review that first-grade list. What fits? What word best describes what you are feeling? Are you angry, sad, or scared? Label the emotion and then tell yourself that the feeling is a valid one. This is not the time for you to find fault with your feelings or challenge your thinking. Simply get in touch with how you feel.

Use this new form for a week, charting your IBS symptoms, the situations in which flare-ups occur, and any relevant emotional reactions. Over the course of time, look to see if there are any patterns. You may be surprised at what you find.

Louis is a twenty-eight-year-old stay-at-home dad whose IBS symptoms became prominent following the birth of his first child. Although he perceived himself to be a fairly confident new parent, due to having spent a lot of time baby-sitting for nieces and nephews, his self-monitoring sheets indicated otherwise. His Feelings column was consistently filled in with worry, anxiety, and doubt. He noticed that these emotions were most prominent in the morning, after his wife left for work. His abdominal distress was also more pronounced around this time. Self-monitoring helped Louis to get in touch with his fears about his ability to take care of his infant the whole day all by himself. Identifying these fears helped Louis to develop positive self-affirmations that reduced his anxiety and significantly relieved his intestinal symptoms.

Self-Monitoring Sheet

Date	Situation	Symptoms	Feelings

Common IBS Emotions

You don't need to reinvent the wheel. Although IBS is a disorder marked by isolation, you know that you are certainly not the only one out there dealing with this. As such, there are emotional reactions that are shared by IBS patients. The discussion of these emotions that follows should help you to fill in your Feelings column.

Dealing with the Diagnosis

Being diagnosed with a chronic illness is bound to touch off a variety of emotions. Believe it or not, some people are actually relieved. Janet is a thirty-five-year-old teacher who told me, "Finally, a doctor was able to tell me what was wrong with me and give it a name! I was so relieved that I started to cry. I was absolutely convinced that I had cancer. It was a great feeling to know that with treatment, my symptoms would become more manageable."

Al was not quite so happy. He was extremely angry that he had developed a disorder that significantly interfered with his ability to do his job as a policeman, a job that he loved. "I have had to take off so many days of work because of this. I'm going crazy just sitting around my house, wondering if I'm ever going to feel better."

Jacqueline was filled with a sense of hopelessness. Her reaction to her IBS diagnosis was, "Nothing has ever been easy for me in my whole life. This is just one more thing. I think happiness is a crock, or just meant for other people." Jacqueline's IBS was complicated by a severe, long-standing depression. For her, a combination of psychotherapy and antidepressant medication helped her to overcome her hopelessness and make some positive changes in her life.

You may be able to relate to some of the above feelings. Other relevant emotions are grief (for the loss of your health), skepticism (maybe the doctors missed something), and anxiety (how bad is this going to get?). You may have your own unique reaction to having IBS. These emotional reactions don't just occur at the time of diagnosis, but may reappear whenever you are symptomatic. Don't just brush off your feelings by saying to yourself, "Other people have worse things happen to them." Although this may be true, being sick is never easy, and you're entitled to react to it.

Fear, Panic, and Anticipatory Anxiety

With IBS, these emotions often become such a part of your everyday functioning that you don't even notice them. As we've discussed before, at times these emotions become so prominent that you would qualify for an anxiety disorder (now that's one heck of a prize, huh?). Although these are all quite similar, with similar effects on your body, there are some important distinctions.

Fear is fairly self-explanatory. We feel afraid when we feel threatened, when we sense that some harm will come to us. Fears can be associated with concerns regarding our own security, the safety of others, or our financial status.

Panic is much more acute and reactive. We panic in the face of a perceived or immediate crisis. The feeling of panic is associated with a strong physiological response and often makes our thinking cloudy.

Anticipatory anxiety is *very* common in IBS. The trauma of getting ill leaves IBS patients prone to worrying about upcoming events and experiences. With anticipatory anxiety you experience the sensation of fear even though you aren't dealing directly with the feared event. Anticipatory anxiety can become so severe that it results in a kind of psychological paralysis.

Just to lighten things up a bit, let me give you a silly example to help you to understand the differences among these three emotions. Let's say that you try out a new restaurant. You notice that the floors are dirty. You fear that the unsanitary conditions will make you sick. Your meal is served and a large bug crawls out. Now you panic. Finally, you develop such anticipatory anxiety that you vow that from now on you will stay home and cook!

Shame and Embarrassment

Like the fear-based emotions, shame and embarrassment may have also become a part of your daily existence. If you suffered from allergies or asthma, you would probably have little difficulty telling others when you aren't feeling well. Disclosing your discomfort opens the door for others to offer you comfort and support. Unfortunately, most people with IBS are not as comfortable talking about their problem because it is embarrassing. When, in the company of others you experience pain, gurgling, and at the very worst actually (oh, I hate to even say it) pass wind, it can be mortifying. Survivable, yes, but mortifying to be sure.

Shame has the added component of self-blame. When we feel ashamed, we are either judging ourselves too harshly or imagining that others are doing so. Keeping your disorder hidden from others only serves to magnify these feelings of shame. As you have done nothing to bring this upon yourself, this negative self-judgment is not only unhelpful, but extremely unfair.

As I worked with one of my patients to reduce her feelings of shame, Deirdre argued with me. "I worry about everything! I know I brought this upon myself. I'm so ashamed. I feel like a failure at life." I told her that I know lots of people who worry about everything but don't have irritable bowel syndrome. Although her excessive worrying didn't help matters, it by no means caused her illness. I told her that she had nothing to be ashamed of and actually should be admired for carrying on so well with her life in spite of the fact that she was coping with a very disruptive chronic illness.

Strategies for Self-Soothing

Remember how it felt to be four years old and to have your mother give you a big hug after you fell down and scraped your knee? Reaching maturity has a lot of advantages, but those kinds of soothing experiences become rare. As an adult, it is now your job to look for opportunities for self-soothing. Some people are very good at this, while others haven't the slightest idea what I'm talking about.

Say "ouch." This doesn't protect you from injury (physical or emotional), but verbalizing your discomfort helps to relieve it. I'm not giving you permission to go around whining or complaining, just saying you should acknowledge within your own head when you have a negative emotional reaction to something. It's okay to say "This really stinks that I have to deal with this IBS stuff. I hate it!" I've cleaned that up a bit—feel free to use whatever language you feel comfortable with.

Normalize your reactions. People are always saying to me, "I know this sounds crazy, but this is how I feel." Your feelings are never crazy. Emotions are by definition not rational, but merely a reflection of your personality and your experiences. Chances are that many other people have also felt the same way, or would if they were in your shoes.

Treat yourself kindly. Become your own best friend. I call this the art of selfishness. If you take care of yourself, you will have much more to give to other people. So many people make the mistake of never putting themselves first and then burn out, which leaves them with nothing to offer anyone else. As you become aware of your emotions (and fill in that Feelings column!), ask yourself what you would say or do to a friend who was feeling that way. If you're afraid, reassure yourself. If you're angry, work to calm yourself down. If you're sad, let yourself cry. Indulge yourself with the things that bring you comfort, within reason of course. Treating yourself doesn't always have to involve food or spending money. A hot bath, a stroll around the neighborhood, and a call to a friend can all be quite soothing. Try a variety of things, and you will find that your efforts go beyond self-soothing and end up enriching your life.

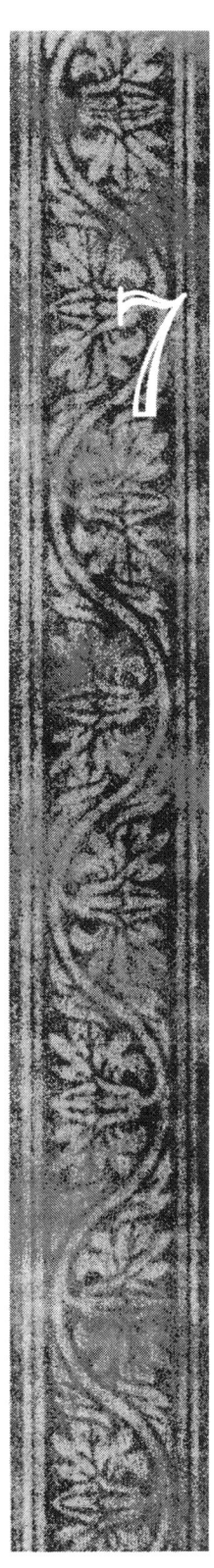

7 MONITORING YOUR THOUGHTS

What's a book about IBS without a good Port-A-Pottie story? A woman was attending a tailgate party before a professional football game. She excused herself to use the Port-A-Pottie. When she came back, she said, "It was disgusting! Someone peed in the pocketbook holder." Her husband said gently, "Honey, there is no such thing as a pocketbook holder in a Port-A-Pottie."

Logic Games

When we react directly to what occurs around us (like being revolted that this woman had for years been placing her pocketbook in urinals), we experience emotions that are manageable and give us information for navigating through our world. However, this process of directly responding is often interrupted by our thought processes which, for a variety of reasons, are not always clear and rational. Our thoughts can be distorted based on our personalities, our emotional state, our past experiences, and lack of information. How we think affects what we feel. If we view situations rationally and reasonably, our emotional responses are healthy and helpful. When our thinking gets distorted, it can lead to unnecessary or overblown emotional responses.

Let me give you an example. Let's say that you begin to experience painful abdominal cramps at a party. If you think, "Oh no, I'm going to be sick. I have got to get out of here right now," you'll end up feeling quite anxious. If, instead, you say to yourself, "Stay calm. See what happens. Maybe the cramps will go away. If not, I'll just excuse myself and use the bathroom. When it's over, I can go back to enjoying the party," you will feel more relaxed and confident about your ability to handle the situation.

Similarly, how we feel can affect what we think. When we're upset, we tend not to think clearly. If we actively work to correct our thinking, we can calm ourselves down and cope more effectively with the upsetting situation.

The relationship among thoughts, feelings, and IBS symptoms is like a logic problem from high school math. If A affects B, and B affects C, then A affects C. If our thoughts affect our emotions, and our emotions affect our gastrointestinal system, then how we think affects our GI system as well. In the above example, if you panic upon experiencing some hint of intestinal distress, you are at risk for setting off your system and maximizing the probability of experiencing severe symptoms. If you think rationally and remain calm, you increase the chances that your intestinal system will calm down and you will feel okay.

Therefore, if you work toward healthier thinking about IBS and your life in general, you will be rewarded with a reduction in IBS symptoms. This notion is supported by research. People who are treated with cognitive therapy, which teaches skills for challenging and modifying faulty thinking, experience relief from their IBS symptoms.

Self-Monitoring

We've talked about faulty thinking in other parts of this book: now it's time to begin to look directly at your thoughts, in order to determine the relationship between the way that you think, the way that you feel, and the way that your body reacts. Your self-monitoring sheets, as shown below, will now be expanded to keep track of what you are thinking in relationship to your IBS symptoms and your emotional reactions. When you are experiencing IBS symptoms and/or emotional upset, try to get in touch with what your thoughts are at the time. Everyone has an internal voice; some people are very much in tune with it, whereas others need to work to pay better attention to it. Ask yourself "What am I thinking?" and "What are my thoughts on this?" Record these under the Thoughts column. We will be discussing ways to identify the thinking mistakes that you are prone to. Once you become aware of them, you can learn to avoid being misled by them into unnecessary upset.

Remember to keep on identifying and labeling your emotional reactions. Knowing how you are feeling will help you to identify your thinking errors. If you are thinking, "I feel that...," the word "that" indicates that whatever is to follow is a thought rather than an emotion. Record it under the Thoughts column. The key to healthy emotional processing is to remember that your emotions are always valid. They might be based on faulty thinking, but they are valid simply because they reflect your reaction to your world. Thoughts are not always valid. They are often based on something other than logic and thus can be challenged and replaced with healthier alternatives, which will result in feelings that are more manageable.

Are You Making These Mistakes?

Illogical thinking is something that we all do, IBS or no IBS. Some of the distortions are due to the way that our brain processes outside stimuli and information. The brain works somewhat like the post office, categorizing and classifying information. And just like at the post office, sometimes data gets misfiled.

Self-Monitoring Sheet

Situation	Symptoms	Feelings	Thoughts

Another way to understand how thinking errors are made is to think about what happens when you play back a homemade videotape or audiotape. Aren't you surprised by the amount of background noise? Our brains automatically filter out stimuli that is deemed unimportant. Similarly, our brains have to filter out and categorize *all* the information that they are presented with. In order to do this, facts get lumped together, at times in ways that aren't always the most helpful. These errors have been labeled in a variety of ways: cognitive distortions, faulty thinking, irrational thoughts. Irrational in this context doesn't mean crazy—it just refers to thoughts that aren't based on rational analysis.

A thought is considered to be irrational if:

1. It is not true.

2. It is not based on logic.

3. There is no evidence to support it.

As you begin to analyze your thoughts, you will consider these conditions and work to change them so that you feel better emotionally and physically. The following discussion will help to acquaint you with some typical thinking errors. Later on in the chapter, we'll also cover some of the most common thinking errors related to IBS.

All-or-Nothing Thinking

In the brain's effort to organize information, it is prone to lumping things together into all-or-nothing, black-and-white, absolutistic thoughts. As we know rationally, the only absolute things in this life are death and taxes. However, we all tend to view other things as being set in stone. "Failing that test will be the worst thing that could happen to me" and "People are all out for themselves" are examples of absolute, all-or-nothing thinking. There are several common cognitive distortions that involve all-or-nothing thinking. We will discuss each in turn.

Shoulds

This is probably going to be the easiest thinking error to identify. The word "should" implies an absolute set of standards for our own behavior and that of others. When we violate this rigid, unrealistic standard, we feel guilty. When we perceive that others have violated these unyielding standards, we feel angry. The problem with the word "should" is that if it really were absolute that people would behave the way we think they should, then they would. However, as we all know, people act in all kinds of goofy ways. To expect anything else doesn't make sense. To walk around with these expectations, only to be constantly upset by the violation of them, leads to a lot of unnecessary anguish. Although it certainly would be better if people acted in a predictable or considerate manner, there is no absolute guarantee that they will. This is the faulty logic on which the word "should" is based.

Never/Always

The use of the words "never" and "always" is another example of all-or-nothing thinking. Again the brain lumps together information in a way that isn't always the most helpful. You may say to someone else, "You're never on time." Odds are that, just by random chance, even the most persistently tardy person sometimes ends up being where they are supposed to be on time. "I always screw up" is an example of the type of thought that leads to feelings of low self-esteem. Again, there are few absolutes in this world, so the use of the words "always" and "never" is rarely warranted.

Perfectionism

Perfectionism involves holding ourselves accountable to unreasonable or unrealistic standards of behavior. This kind of thinking presupposes that horrible things will happen if we don't live up to these standards. "If my house isn't immaculate, my friends will judge me and not like me." Perfectionism results in chronic anxiety, tension, and pressure, as one attempts to meet arbitrary, unrealistic goals.

Awfulizing

Ah, here's something you might be familiar with. This is the tendency to view something that is bad as absolutely awful. Thus all bad things are thrown together into the same horrible stewpot, without any differentiation as to how bad they might be. There are certainly bad things in this world, but we tend to throw around words like awful, horrible, and terrible when they aren't really justified. Besides the fact that most things aren't really that bad, the use of these words interferes with our ability to focus on our own competence in dealing with difficult situations.

Labeling

This cognitive error has to do with applying labels to ourselves and others. The problem with this is that people can't be defined in a word. A negative label engenders emotional responses that aren't necessarily warranted. For example, negative self-talk such as "Oh, I'm such a loser" results in feelings of low self-confidence. When a label is applied to others, e.g. "You're a self-centered pig," it makes the other person feel angry and defensive. And even the most self-centered pig, on occasion, might be known to do something thoughtful.

Fortune-Telling

In addition to all-or-nothing thinking errors, people are often prone to the belief that they can predict the future. This kind of fortune-telling goes on constantly, but most people are unaware that they are doing it. An example of fortune-telling would be "I just know that I'm going to be physically miserable if I go to work today." If you truly had the ability to accurately predict what was going to happen in the future, you would be a millionaire, because you would have used your talents to pick the correct numbers in the lottery.

Anxious projection into the future is similar to fortune-telling; you just phrase the worry differently, using the words "What if. . . ?" Although it sounds like you're just thinking about a possible happenstance, you are actually reacting emotionally, as if the feared situation is already upon you. The main problem with fortune-telling, projection, and "what if" thinking is that in this unpredictable world, we really never know what will happen. The thoughts create anxiety, but no helpful coping strategies get kicked in, because you haven't yet gotten to the river that you need to cross. Anxious projection wastes the resources that you need to cope with difficult situations. The antidote to all of this is planning, which involves thinking about what is likely to happen and preparing yourself to handle the difficulties of the upcoming stressful situation.

Mind Reading

Like fortune-telling, this is a circus trick that many of us do all day long, even though it's pointless. We constantly make assumptions about what other people are thinking, and as if that weren't bad enough, our assumption is generally that the other person is thinking something negative about us. "Because my children are acting up, those people must think I'm a terrible parent." Most of the time, other people are so worried about the impression that they're making on you that they don't have time to pass judgment. Now, some people *are* critical and judgmental in their thinking. (Some of these people don't even have the good sense to keep these thoughts to themselves.) If the other person truly falls into that category, you might not want to make their opinion so important, because they aren't very nice anyway.

The other common mind-reading mistake is to assume that others are mad at us if we sense that something is bothering them. You may be tempted to make the fatal mistake of asking, "Are you mad at me?" If they weren't mad at you to begin with, they might be now, and you may find yourself the unwitting victim of someone else's bad mood. If the other person is upset with you, it is their responsibility to tell you so that things can be worked out. If they don't choose to do this, then it's their loss. If you feel compelled to ask anything, a good approach is to say, "You look upset. Is something the matter? Would you like to talk about it?" This opens the door for communication, but without setting you up for use as a scapegoat.

Finding Connections

You now know that there's a direct connection between types of cognitive distortions and unhealthy or overblown emotional responses. You have already been working to try to better identify and label your feelings. This skill will help you to pinpoint the thinking errors that you might be prone to. If you can't quite figure out what you're thinking, figure out how you're feeling, and see if you are making the thinking error that is usually associated with that particular emotion.

Depression

When we're feeling depressed, our thoughts are usually very all-or-nothing, with a negative view of ourselves, the world, and the future. We think things like "Things will never get any better," "I'll always be stuck in some dead-end job," and "There's never any justice in this crazy world." The problem with this type of negative thinking is that these statements are simply not true. Just because a person is going through a difficult time doesn't automatically mean that these problems are forever.

When we direct these negative absolute thoughts at ourselves, we experience feelings of low self-esteem. A good example of this type of thought is, "I must be a weak person, because I can't even handle life without running to a bathroom all the time." If you are feeling depressed or down on yourself, look for the cognitive errors of all-or-nothing thinking, labeling, and awfulizing.

Guilt

Guilt comes from those "shoulds." We think that we should be perfect, that we *should* be able to be all things to all people, and that it's our job to prevent others from ever experiencing a negative emotion. If you're feeling guilty, look for shoulds, musts, and perfectionist thoughts.

A common refrain is, "They made me feel guilty." But only you can make yourself feel guilty, by choosing to buy what the other person is selling. For their own purposes, it's very convenient for another person to tell you that you're not doing the right thing. It's up to you to decide if what the other person is asking of you is reasonable. If not, you have nothing to feel guilty about.

Along the same lines, don't automatically feel guilty just because someone around you is upset. Other people need to take responsibility for their reactions to what you do. If you feel that you acted in a reasonable manner, but the other person takes offense, you might want to consider what it is about them that caused the upset. Are they overly sensitive, or do they have unrealistic expectations for the behavior of others? To defuse such a situation, you may want to express your regret that they're upset but you don't necessarily have to feel guilty for upsetting them.

Anger

The maladaptive thoughts involved in excessive or prolonged anger have to do with "shoulds" for the behavior of ourselves and others and the absolute thought of "It's not fair!" We feel angry at ourselves or at other people when there is a violation of our internally defined list of "shoulds." "He should never have cut in front of us like that! How dare he?" Well, if it were so absolute that he shouldn't do it, he wouldn't have done it. And, how dare he—well he just did, didn't he? The world is filled with all types of behavior, not just the civilized behavior that we expect and desire.

The thought that the world should be fair gets us into a lot of trouble and results in a lot of unhealthy anger. The world has been operating for centuries without a guarantee of fairness and justice. Although good-hearted and well-intentioned people do try to impose justice, the very nature of humans is that life will be filled with a lot of inequity. Thus, a more reasonable expectation is that things will at times be unfair. It is far better to cope with this fact rather than to expend a lot of energy protesting it.

Anxiety

If you're feeling anxious, your most likely cognitive errors are projection and awfulizing. Projection, as you know, involves thinking about the worst-case scenario as if it were a given. It's not too hard to see how that would make you feel anxious, tense, and jumpy. Awfulizing makes us feel anxious because we think that whatever it is that we have to face will be absolutely terrible, and we'll be unable to cope.

Awfulizing and projection leave us at risk for contributing to a self-fulfilling prophecy. A self-fulfilling prophecy is one in which we determine ahead of time what the outcome is going to be, and then unwittingly make decisions that lead us in that particular direction. With anxiety, a self-fulfilling prophecy works like this: You anticipate that you'll be anxious in an upcoming situation. This heightens your attention to signs of anxiety, your fight-or-flight reflex is turned on, and, lo and behold, you end up feeling anxious. For example, when IBS is a factor, your anxiety may trigger the very same intestinal symptoms that you predicted you would suffer in a particular situation.

Shame

Shame results from all-or-nothing thoughts regarding acceptable human behavior. Like the "shoulds," the set of standards is arbitrary and doesn't account for the wide variability inherent in humanity. Shame also usually involves mind reading, as you assume that others are judging you harshly for whatever norm you feel you have violated.

Labeling also rears its ugly head in the experience of shame. We may label ourselves a freak, a sinner, or a pervert, or we think that others have done so. We make the mistake of coloring our whole personhood based on one small fact about ourselves. But when people look at others, they don't generally think that way. People usually form an overall opinion of someone, either positive or negative. One perceived misstep, whether it be someone making a major error at work, having too much to drink, or passing wind in public, is not usually enough to change that overall opinion.

Common Irrational Thoughts about IBS

As you work to identify your irrational thoughts, it may be helpful to read about the kinds of cognitive mistakes that many IBS patients make. Some of them may be familiar to you, others may help you discover the roots of your anxious reactions, and certain ones may make you realize how silly we humans can sometimes be.

"It would be absolutely terrible if I got sick when others are around to see." Here's a good example of awfulizing. Getting sick is certainly unpleasant, but it is far from one of the more tragic things that could happen to a person. This thought also implies a little mind reading, as it makes the assumption that others would think poorly of you if you were to show signs of being ill in their presence.

"I'm only assured of feeling well if I stay at home." This thought reflects all-or-nothing thinking, as it maintains a guarantee of freedom from symptoms if one never goes out. As we know, there are no real guarantees in life. The implied irrational thought, *"If I go out, I just know that I'll get sick, and that will be unbearable,"* exemplifies fortune-telling and is a self-fulfilling prophecy regarding what would happen if one were to venture out. The tail end of that thought can be categorized as awfulizing.

"Only certain foods are safe." People with IBS are at risk for all-or-nothing thinking regarding food. Their symptoms may be triggered by a variety of factors (e.g. hormones, stress), yet they attribute the outbreak to whatever food they just ate. The very real and dangerous risk of this type of "bad food" labeling is that the individual ends up with a very narrow, restricted, nutrient-deficient diet.

"My IBS symptoms are completely unpredictable and unmanageable." Besides being an example of all-or-nothing, absolutistic thinking, it is simply not true that IBS symptoms are unpredictable. Once you learn to identify triggers, you'll be better able to understand when and how your IBS is likely to manifest itself, and you'll be better equipped to deal with unpleasant symptoms.

"What if I don't make it to a bathroom in time?" It's not too hard to figure out that this is an example of "What if" anxious projection. The underlying implication is that this would be an unbearable, unsurvivable event.

"Other people are going to think that I'm abnormal (weak, strange) because I'm always running to the bathroom." Mind reading and labeling are at play here. Remember: No one really knows what another person is thinking. In addition, in this wacky world you have to do a lot more than just run to the bathroom to earn the label of strange. A related cognition, *"People are going to think that I'm crazy, that it's all in my head, or that I'm making it up for attention,"* suffers from the same cognitive errors of mind reading and labeling.

"My whole life is ruined by IBS. I will always be miserable because of it." This all-or-nothing statement assumes that because of one decidedly miserable disorder, your whole life need be miserable. You're also fortune-telling that today's discomfort is going to be forever.

"The doctor must be missing something. I can't be this sick and not have a life-threatening disease." This thought is just plain old irrational because there is no evidence to support it. IBS can be diagnosed with confidence just based on your symptom picture. If your symptoms, test results, and your doctor's diagnosis don't indicate the presence of a more serious disorder, then to think otherwise is to be giving airtime in your head to a thought that is simply not true.

Self-Monitoring in Action

Margaret was a twenty-year-old college student when she first came into treatment. Her IBS first manifested itself in the second semester of her junior year. Besides there being a family history of IBS, it appeared that her symptoms were so severe at this point in her life due to her excessive focus on getting a job in the finance world following graduation the following year. Her self-monitoring sheets give a good illustration of a variety of cognitive errors.

Margaret's Self-Monitoring Sheet

Situation	Symptoms	Feelings	Thoughts
Thinking about going out to dinner w/ roommate	Cramping, diarrhea - 5	Anxiety!	There is no way that I am leaving this room! How can I enjoy dinner if I will be so sick? (Fortune-telling)
Preparing for exam	Cramps, diarrhea - 5	Anxiety	I have to do well on this exam or my grade point average will never be good enough for me to get a good internship. (Perfectionism, Fortune-telling)
Taking Calculus exam	Cramps, gas pains - 5	Anxiety	This is a nightmare! What if I have to run to the bathroom? My professor will never let me. (Awfulizing, Projection, Mind Reading)
Talking with mother on phone	Tense, stomach in knots - 3	Angry, upset	She doesn't understand. She thinks I'm just doing this for attention. She should know better. She's always running to the bathroom whenever she's stressed. (Should, Mind Reading)

Margaret's worksheet shows that she is fairly stressed out. She is applying too much pressure on herself to establish a career, when right now she would be better served by just focusing on doing her best in her current courses. Her tendency toward future projection is resulting in a high anxiety level and exacerbating her physical symptoms. She also needs work in therapy to learn how to better assert her needs and get help from others. Her inability to access needed support was evidenced by her self-monitoring sheets, with her fear of asking her professor to excuse her so that she could go to the bathroom, and the frustration she experienced in her phone call with her mother.

Identifying Your Irrationality

You should now have a fairly good idea about the types of cognitive errors that contribute to unhealthy emotional reactions. The next step is to learn to identify and label your irrational thoughts as such. This will be your first step in reducing the intensity of negative emotions, as you will no longer just be automatically reacting to your thinking.

Take a red pen or a yellow highlighter and go through your self-monitoring sheets. Look for examples of cognitive distortions and underline them. (This is what I do when a patient of mine brings in their sheets.) The Thoughts column gives me invaluable information about the way that each individual patient views the world. Identifying the cognitive distortions helps me to quickly pinpoint areas for intervention.

Try to figure out which category your irrational thoughts fall into. Are you mind reading, fortune-telling, shoulding? Categorizing the thoughts will help you to challenge and replace them, skills we'll be discussing in the next chapter.

As you look over your self-monitoring sheets, do you see any patterns between your thoughts and your IBS symptoms? When you predict that you'll be ill, do you work yourself up into such a state that you end up feeling miserable? Do you put so much pressure on yourself to show a perfect facade to the world that you end up making yourself sick? Are your expectations of others so unreasonable that you find yourself chronically angry and tense, with your stomach tied in knots? Is there a direct relationship between what you think, how you feel emotionally, and how you feel physically? There usually is, and this gives you plenty of work space for reducing your symptoms, feeling healthy, and regaining the freedom to enjoy your life.

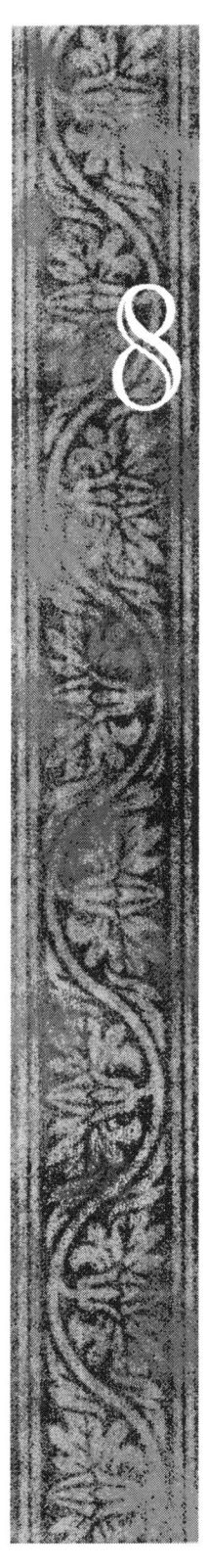

8 A Calm Mind in a Calm Body

Congratulations. You've now achieved a level of self-awareness that many people lack. No longer at the mercy of your immediate knee-jerk reaction to the world, you've successfully acquired the ability to stand back and evaluate your perceptions before automatically responding to them.

It's now time to take it to the next level. You'll learn how to challenge your unhealthy ways of thinking and develop healthy, adaptive thoughts. These thoughts will help you to remain calm, which will have the added benefit of keeping your body, especially your intestinal system, calm as well. You know that great feeling of having enough conscious control to change the story of a nightmare so that it has a happy ending? Think about how different you feel when you wake up. Challenging and replacing your irrational thoughts is a little bit like that. If you change the way that you think about a situation, your feelings become more manageable. Although at first this may take a bit of work, with practice it will start to happen automatically.

When it comes to healthy emotional processing, you already have the first two steps down pat. You have been practicing labeling and validating your emotions and looking for cognitive distortions. From here you will learn to challenge your irrational thoughts and replace them with a healthier perspective. This will leave you with emotions that are at a workable level, useful for either problem solving or self-soothing.

The Challenge

Once you have identified a thought, it's time to establish whether it is a true, logical response to the given situation, or an irrational or distorted one. This involves asking the following questions:

1. Is this thought true?

2. Is there evidence to support this thought?

3. Does this thought really make sense?

If the answer to any of these questions is "no," then you probably have an irrational thought on your hands. The task then becomes to replace the thought with one that is more logical and has evidence to support it. This replacement thought will then result in a manageable, helpful level of emotionality. To come up with a replacement thought, ask yourself:

1. What would be a logical way to think about this situation?

2. What conclusion *can* be drawn from the evidence?

3. If I think about this objectively, what makes the most sense?

Let me give you an example of how this works. Let's take a thought like, "Everyone thinks that this IBS is all in my head." The words "everyone" and "all" indicate that this is an example of all-or-nothing thinking, as well as some mind reading. Question the thought: "Is it true that my IBS is all in my head?" No, of course not; there is ample research to support a physiological basis for irritable bowel syndrome. "Is there evidence to support the notion that everyone else thinks it's all in my head?" No, in fact, the medical community at large acknowledges that IBS is an identifiable, diagnosable disorder. You probably also have *some* friends who understand and are able to offer support to you in your efforts to cope with IBS. If not, the problem is not that no one takes you seriously, but that you need new friends. Given all this evidence, does it make sense to continue to torture yourself with the belief that everyone thinks that you're making too big a deal out of this or just looking for attention?

Now that you've challenged the thought, you need to come up with a healthy replacement. What is a logical way to think about this particular issue? Although it may be true that some ignorant individuals might question the veracity of your disorder, evidence exists to support your position. What conclusion can be drawn from the evidence? It's clear that IBS is an intestinal disorder in which there is a physiological basis for a hyperreactivity of the intestines to outside stimuli. If you think about this objectively, what makes the most sense? You should avoid ignorant, unhelpful people, seek out support from kind, helpful, understanding individuals, and stop questioning your own judgment about your very real physical distress.

Rebut and Replace

When a person experiences an unhealthy emotional reaction, there are several cognitive distortions that are likely to be underlying contributors. We'll take a look at some of the core thoughts that are behind these feelings to help you to establish your own repertoire of challenges and replacements. Although thoughts specific to your own personality and way of reacting to the world may not show up in the following discussion, there are likely to be some that come close. People seem so different on the surface due to a wide variability in their behavioral responses, but there tends to be some similarity in the way that people think when experiencing a particular emotion. Thus, the following thoughts are likely to manifest themselves in a variety of different circumstances.

Depression

When people are depressed, their thoughts tend to be quite negative, with a bleak view of themselves, the world, and their future. We'll take an example of each one of these in turn.

Thought: I'm such a loser, I never do anything right.

Distortion: All-or-nothing thinking, never/always, labeling

Challenge: Is it really true that I never do *anything* right?

Replacement: Like everyone else, I have my weaknesses and I make mistakes. I also have a lot of strengths and talents, even if it's difficult to focus on them right now.

Thought: Bad things always happen to me. The world just seems to have it in for me.

Distortion: Always/never, personalization

Challenge: Is there really any evidence that the world has singled you out to make your life miserable?

Replacement: Sure, bad things have happened to me, but they happen to a lot of people. Life is random, and I have to admit that I have also been given some good things in my life, as well.

Thought: I guess I'm just meant to be miserable forever.

Distortion: All-or-nothing thinking, fortune-telling

Challenge: Where is the evidence to support the notion that I'm meant to be miserable forever?

Replacement: There might be some evidence that, for right now, I'm feeling pretty lousy, but there is no way for me to accurately predict what will happen to me down the road, unless I make my misery a self-fulfilling prophecy.

Guilt

Guilt comes from unreasonable expectations for ourselves, expectations that don't take into account the fact that we're human. There is usually an underlying "should." Also watch out for taking full responsibility for something that perhaps someone else had a part in. Ask yourself, "Do I have control?" If you don't have control, you aren't responsible.

Thought:	It's all my fault that that person got so upset. I should have known better.
Distortion:	All-or-nothing thinking regarding blame, should
Challenge:	Is it true that it really was only my fault that the other person reacted the way that they did? Does the evidence support the fact that I should have known better?
Replacement:	If I had known ahead of time that this was a sore spot for this particular individual, I never would have said anything. I have to acknowledge that this person got upset, not just because of what I said, but because of how they chose to respond to it. I regret the fact that they did get upset, and I will now know better in the future how this person is likely to respond.

Anger

With anger, it's important to make sure that you aren't "shoulding" on others, or making yourself crazy over the fact that the world isn't fair.

Thought:	They had no right to do that! They should have known better.
Distortion:	All-or-nothing thinking, should
Challenge:	Does it make sense to say that they had no right to do what they did, when in actuality, people are free to behave in any way that they choose? If it were so true that they should have known better, wouldn't they have acted accordingly?
Replacement:	People can act any way they want. In fact, they act like knuckleheads all the time. I also don't have to like what they did, but I don't have to make myself crazy because they violated one of the rules according to me.
Thought:	It is so unfair that they did what they did and then walked away scot-free.
Distortion:	All-or-nothing thinking regarding fairness

Challenge:	Where is the evidence that this world is a fair place?
Replacement:	I don't like what they did, but I don't need to make it worse for myself by focusing on the fact that they seem to be getting away with it. In fact, I don't really know for sure that there won't be some negative consequences somewhere along the line for this person for this offense.

Anxiety

When you're feeling anxious, keep in mind that you are most likely responding to thoughts in your head, rather than an immediate crisis situation. This type of anxiety reaction uses up valuable resources for coping with real emergencies or difficult situations. Look for projection and "what if" thoughts. Remember to think about probability and perspective. How likely is it that the feared event will become a reality? How bad is it really, in the overall scheme of things?

Thought:	Oh, God, what if that happened? I would never be able to cope with it.
Distortion:	"What if," implied awfulizing, always/never
Challenge:	Do I really know for sure what's going to happen? Where is the evidence that I'll be unable to cope with whatever happens?
Replacement:	Let me wait and see what's really going to happen. Even if the worst happens, although it might be bad, it is certainly not going to be the end of the world. In any case, I am a competent person, and I'll be able to handle whatever comes up. I may not handle it perfectly, but I certainly will survive it.
Thought:	I just know that's going to happen. It would be absolutely awful.
Distortion:	Fortune-telling, awfulizing
Challenge:	Do I really have the ability to predict the future? Is it really true that it would be the most awful thing that could happen?

Replacement: It makes no sense for me to be dealing with this now, because there is no way for me to know what's really going to happen. Let me cross that bridge when I get to it. Even if it's difficult to cope with, I need to remember that there are worse things that happen in this world.

Shame

In my practice, I have come across such unnecessary shame. People experience so much distress because they hold themselves accountable for something over which they have no control, or because they don't forgive themselves for having acted in a human, fallible way. The main cognitive errors involved in the experience of shame have to do with holding rigid, inflexible views regarding appropriate human behavior and regarding other people's judgment of that behavior. Secrecy is often deemed essential to the ashamed person, yet it is in secrecy that the feelings of shame flourish. Exposing your shame-related cognitions to the light of day, or to a sympathetic person, can help to decrease the hold that these thoughts have on your self-worth.

Thought: I am a horrible person because I did that.

Distortion: Labeling, awfulizing, implied should

Challenge: Does it make sense to make a judgment about the whole of me based on one thing that I did? Were there extenuating circumstances? Was I completely in control of the situation?

Replacement: I need to remember that, like everyone else, I am human. This one thing doesn't negate all of the nice things about me. I need to forgive myself and move on.

Thought: If anyone ever found out about this, I would die of embarrassment. I would never be able to show my face again.

Distortion: Implied awfulizing, implied mind reading and labeling, always/never

Challenge: Is it really true that it would be the end of the world if someone were to find out? Is there any evidence that anyone ever died from embarrassment?

Replacement: While I might prefer to keep this to myself, I need to remember that it wouldn't kill me if someone were to find out. If someone else's opinion of me would be changed by just one thing, rather than the whole of me, maybe it's not good for me to be around that person.

Healthy Emotional Processing

Let's take a moment to review the step-by-step process for dealing with your emotions in a healthy, helpful manner:

1. Label and validate the emotion.

2. Identify the underlying thoughts.

3. Look for cognitive distortions.

4. If distortions exist, challenge them and develop healthy replacement thoughts.

5. Use the resulting emotion as a stimulus for problem solving or self-soothing.

The skills you've just developed will help you in many ways. First of all, these skills will help you to reduce emotional triggers for IBS symptoms. They will also help you deal with living a life affected by a chronic illness. Most importantly, well-developed emotional processing skills are essential for overall mental health.

An Illustration

Diane is a forty-two-year-old bookkeeper for an exclusive private school. She entered into therapy when she experienced such severe anxiety about riding on a train that she was unable to go to work. She explained to me that several months earlier, she grew quite ill on the train, experiencing such severe nausea, vomiting, and weakness that she had to ask a fellow passenger to get her some help. The train was stopped at the next station until an ambulance arrived to take Diane to a hospital. Diane reported that she found the whole experience extremely stressful. She felt very vulnerable because she had to rely on strangers for aid. She was mortified that the entire train had to be held up because of her distress.

While she was in the hospital, Diane was diagnosed with gallbladder disease and underwent surgery to have her gallbladder removed. When she came to see me, she had recovered from the operation but was terrified about getting back on the train. Our first few sessions consisted of relaxation training and gradual exposure to train rides. This proved successful and she was able to resume commuting to her job.

Although she had reduced her anxiety enough to get on the train, she remained quite anxious throughout the ride and was hypervigilant about physical symptoms. This anxiety appeared to set off her intestinal system and she would end up with cramps and diarrhea; she often spent a large portion of the ride in the train bathroom, which was apparently not a very pleasant place. Due to her continued difficulty, I assigned her the task of self-monitoring her anxiety-producing cognitions.

A review of Diane's self-monitoring sheets indicated that she experienced feelings of panic whenever she thought about getting incapacitated on the train. Underlying the panic was a lot of "what if" and awfulizing. Her biggest fear came from the thought, "If I get sick, I won't be in control, and something terrible could happen to me." My first challenge was, "Where is the evidence that if you got sick you wouldn't be able to take care of yourself?" It was easy to point out to her that her own traumatic experience disproved the thinking behind her biggest fear. She *had* gotten sick, in a public place, surrounded by strangers. She was able to access appropriate, safe care by asking those around her to summon the conductor. In spite of becoming ill, she *was* able to successfully manage the situation and get her needs (for safety and medical treatment) met. She replied, "Well, what if I passed out?" My question was, "What is the probability that you would lose consciousness without any warning?" I informed her that people rarely lose consciousness without some warning, which would provide her with the opportunity to ask for help. I also pointed out to her that it is a natural human tendency to come to the aid of a person in distress. Thus the probability is pretty high that were she to pass out in public, other passengers would alert the authorities, thus ensuring her safety.

Following this discussion, Diane was a lot calmer in response to gastrointestinal symptoms experienced while riding the train. She reminds herself that although getting ill on the train would be an unpleasant experience, and certainly not one she would want to repeat, she *could* count on herself and others to ensure her safety.

Exercise: Cognitive Challenging

On your self-monitoring sheets, you have been recording the thoughts that appear in relationship to your IBS symptoms. You can use the worksheet below to help you develop healthy replacement thoughts. Write down one of your identified thoughts. Look for cognitive distortions and apply the challenge questions from earlier in this chapter. Then fill in the Replacement column with thoughts that more accurately relate to the situation at hand.

Taking the time to write down the healthy thinking that you have come up with will help to strengthen those thoughts for you. At first it may take some work to develop healthy replacement thoughts, but with practice and reinforcement they will come to you more automatically. You will also find that there are similarities in your reaction to various situations, therefore replacement thoughts will be applicable to a variety of circumstances.

Cognitive Challenging Worksheet

Irrational Thought	Challenge	Replacement

Replacement Thoughts

In order to help you to fill out your cognitive challenging worksheets, let's take a look at some of the irrational thoughts that we discussed in the last chapter as being fairly universal for people who experience IBS. The replacement thoughts that follow may be of help to you.

Thought: It would be absolutely terrible if I got sick when others were around to see.

Challenge: Would it really be the worst thing in the world if my IBS became known to others?

Replacement: Although it wouldn't be pleasant to be sick in public, it isn't the worst thing that could happen. People will be supportive and sympathetic, and I can cope with the discomfort until it passes.

Thought: I am only assured of feeling well if I stay home.

Challenge: Where is the evidence that IBS is related to geography?

Replacement: The best way for me to stay well is to stay calm. It is my anxiety setting off my system that increases my chances of being sick, not where I am. It is good for me to get out. I will feel healthier physically and emotionally if I take the steps to enjoy my life.

Thought: If I go out, I just know that I'll get sick, and that would be unbearable.

Challenge: Where is the evidence that I can predict the future?

Replacement: I don't know for sure that I will get sick if I go out. There are steps that I can take to keep my anxiety low, so that I minimize the risk of getting ill. Even if I do get sick, I will just cope with it and be proud of myself for making the attempt to resume my life.

Thought: Only certain foods are safe.

Challenge: Do I really have evidence that so many foods are setting off my IBS? Is it possible that it isn't the food, but the way I'm reacting to certain situations?

Replacement:	Food intolerances are very rare. I do know that at some times, I have difficulty with some food. Therefore I do need to practice caution when I am under stress, but I don't need to overly restrict my diet, which could be detrimental to my overall health.
Thought:	My IBS symptoms are completely unpredictable and unmanageable.
Challenge:	Is it really true that I have no idea when or where my IBS will act up?
Replacement:	I know that there are certain identifiable triggers for IBS symptoms. My self-monitoring sheets will help me to get a grip on them. Once I learn to identify these triggers, then I can work to reduce the impact they have on my health.
Thought:	What if I don't make it to the bathroom on time?
Challenge:	Where is the evidence that I won't get there in time to avoid a problem?
Replacement:	I have to remember that having an accident is an extremely rare occurrence. If I stay calm, I will be able to reduce the urgency and will ensure that I make it to a bathroom.
Thought:	Other people are going to think that I'm abnormal, weak, or strange, because I'm always running to the bathroom.
Challenge:	How is it possible for me to really know what another person is thinking?
Replacement:	There is no way to know for sure what goes on in anybody's head. I have to remember that most people are nice and thus would feel sympathy toward someone who appears to be in distress. People will judge me based on the kind of person that I am, not on how often I go the bathroom.
Thought:	People are going to think that I'm crazy, that it's all in my head, or that I'm making it up just to get attention.

Challenge:	Again, how is it possible for me to know what other people are thinking?
Replacement:	First of all, it isn't healthy for me to be so concerned about what others think. I know that I have a medically recognized disorder. If other people choose to see it otherwise, I don't have to let that be my problem.
Thought:	My whole life is ruined by IBS. I will always be miserable because of it.
Challenge:	Where is the evidence that today's distress will last forever?
Replacement:	It's up to me how much I let this disorder affect my life. I can learn to work to better prevent and manage distressing symptoms, so that I can have a full life in spite of my IBS. It is a disorder that tends to wax and wane, so that even if I am having difficulty now, I need to remember that I will experience episodes of remission.
Thought:	The doctors must have missed something. I can't be this sick and not have a life-threatening disease.
Challenge:	Where is the evidence that I have something other than IBS?
Replacement:	I need to focus on the fact that I don't have the symptoms of any other disease. IBS can make me feel very bad but it doesn't mean that I'm going to die from it.

Calming Self-Talk

Calming self-talk is just what it sounds like. Talking to yourself doesn't mean that you're crazy—in fact, it's a great way to stay sane. Calming self-talk is a strategy for reducing anxiety by talking to yourself in a calm, rational manner regarding the things that usually set off your anxiety. As you fill out your cognitive challenging worksheets, you are providing yourself with a wealth of options to use for calming self-talk. If that little voice inside your head were to keep repeating the words written on the right side of your page, rather than the left, you'd be a lot better off. Keep your replacement thoughts handy, so you can pull them out and look at them whenever you feel anxious about your IBS.

Here are a few handy, calming self-statements:

1. IBS is uncomfortable, but it isn't going to kill me.
2. The calmer I keep myself, the quieter my intestines will be.
3. If I get sick in public, it won't be the end of the world. I will cope with it and get through it.
4. I will find access to a bathroom and my body will cooperate until I get there.
5. If my stomach rumbles or I pass gas, it isn't such a big deal. It happens to everyone at one time or another.
6. Other people will most likely be supportive and understanding, not judgmental and critical.
7. IBS doesn't mean that I'm a weak person. The fact that I can cope with something like this actually points to my strength.

Exercise: Coping Skills Column

You've graduated to a new and improved self-monitoring sheet, which will be the final edition. Note that a new column, Coping Skills, has been added. You have some newly acquired techniques at your disposal that you can now proudly record in this last column. You have learned:

- how to identify cognitive distortions
- cognitive challenging
- replacement thinking
- calming self-talk

In this last column, you can record which of the above options that you used in coping with IBS symptoms and unhelpful emotional reactions. If you would prefer, you can write the specific replacement thoughts and calming self-statements you used, in order to further reinforce this healthier way of thinking. You will be pleased to find that as your Coping Skills column fills up, your record of IBS symptoms will begin to show a decrease in the frequency, intensity, and duration of your distress. Good work. Feeling better is what this is all about.

Self-Monitoring Sheet

Situation	Symptoms	Feelings	Thoughts	Coping Skills

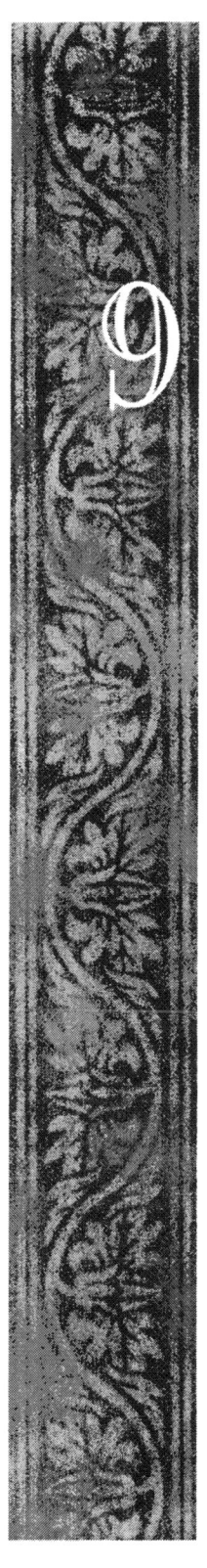

9 THE PROACTIVE APPROACH: BUILDING SKILLS AND BREAKING FREE

You can do anything! That's a bit of a sweeping statement to be sure, but with determination, persistence, practice, and a little bit of luck, a person can do almost anything they set their mind to. People have climbed mountains, written beautiful poetry, grown prize-winning gardens. All it takes is to set a goal and then, as they say, just do it! It's easy to avoid learning a new skill or venturing into unknown territory by thinking, "Oh, that's something I could never do. That's something only a special kind of person could do." But there is absolutely no reason why you could not be that special kind of person. A very regular person named Carolyn McCarthy, who had for years been a very ordinary homemaker, put one foot in front of the other and wound up being elected to the United States House of Representatives. She did have strong motivation, as she committed herself to the issue of gun control after her husband was killed and her son seriously injured by a gunman on a suburban train. I'm sure if a psychic had predicted five years prior to her election that she would someday be a congresswoman, she would have scoffed at the idea. But given a good reason, she took a risk and met with success.

Learning new skills for better management of your IBS need not be quite so dramatic. I just don't want you to read about the steps you could be taking to feel better, and think to yourself, "Oh, that's not for me. I could never learn to be more relaxed," or "Oh, I could never speak up like that, I'm just not that kind of person." Although we don't always have control over how we feel, we do have control over how we choose to act. Certain ways of behaving will help you feel better, just as clearly as certain ways of behaving contribute to feelings of misery. This chapter will teach you, step by step, how to relax your body, deal more effectively with other people, and venture back out into the world with your irritable bowel. Take the risk to try out these skills, and you will gain pride in your accomplishments, feel that you are back in control of your life, and break the confines of IBS.

Develop Relaxation Skills

"Just relax. You'll be fine." Don't you hate it when people say this to you? It's usually right before some kind of harrowing experience, like childbirth or a roller-coaster ride. If only it were that simple to just relax. The ability to relax is a skill, and as with other skills, with practice you can become quite proficient at it. Learning to relax your body is a powerful tool against anxiety. For a person who suffers from IBS, the ability to relax their body, reducing the physical arousal that comes with tension and anxiety might mean the difference between spending time doing something enjoyable and spending time locked in the nearest rest room.

Many people walk through their days with an enormous amount of physical tension and anxiety, which is usually not even in their consciousness. Having a body this tense puts unnecessary strain on various muscle groups and the skeletal structure. With a high anxiety baseline, it doesn't take much to set off the fight-or-flight reflex, resulting in unpleasant physical manifestations of panic. If you have IBS, you know all too well what that means!

Relaxation exercises have two major benefits. Utilizing the exercises on a regular basis lowers your overall anxiety level, leaving you with better resistance to the slings and arrows of life. I liken it to the way boxers conduct themselves during a match. In between punches, boxers work hard to keep themselves loose and relaxed. They bounce on the balls of their feet, jiggle their arms, and try to keep their muscles as relaxed as possible. When they throw a punch, they then focus their energy, tighten up their muscles, and pow! The purpose of keeping themselves loose is so that they aren't burning up their stored resources, but saving them for when it counts, when they want to land a punch. Learn from the pros and work to keep your body as loose and relaxed as possible, saving your energy and resources for the times you really need them. You will find that this has a tremendous impact on your physical health and your overall sense of well-being.

The other benefit of learning relaxation exercises is that they can be used on the spot when you are experiencing an anxiety spike. We have talked about the fight-or-flight mechanism as being like a home security system. When a person has an anxiety disorder or a stress-related illness like IBS, the alarm trigger is sometimes too sensitive, resulting in terror reactions to situations that aren't life threatening. Relaxation exercises provide you with a handy "off" switch. Instead of responding with panic when you first feel those early stirrings or rumbles from your abdomen, you can work to actively reduce your arousal by relaxing your mind and body and turning off the alarm. This is a powerful tool with the remarkable effect of restoring your peace of mind, as you are no longer strictly at the mercy of your intestinal system.

There are a variety of relaxation strategies, and people tend to respond differently to various methods. I like to present my patients with three different components: calming visualization, deep breathing, and progressive muscle relaxation. They then usually select the strategies that work best for them. Try them all and see which are the most comfortable, workable, and helpful for you. You may find that when practicing at home you are able to fully enjoy the benefits of all three, while on the spot, a quick run-through of just one strategy is all you need. I'll give you step-by-step instructions for each component, but if you prefer, there is the option of purchasing commercially prepared relaxation tapes which are readily available at most book and music stores.

When you practice, pick out a spot in your home that is quiet, peaceful, and comfortable. I don't recommend practicing in bed, as the goal is to teach you how to relax, not how to sleep! That ability wouldn't serve you well at your next board meeting or family function. If you have difficulty sleeping, do your relaxation exercises before getting into bed. It's much easier to put a relaxed body to sleep than a tense one. Try to do the exercises at least two times a day, spending approximately twenty minutes enjoying the pleasure of feeling totally relaxed.

Exercise: Calming Visualization

Simply imagining yourself in a quiet, peaceful place can be a great aid toward relaxation. The main benefit of this kind of visualization is that it serves to divert attention away from worrisome thoughts. With practice, just thinking about your quiet place can become a cue for your body to assume a relaxed state, which will result in a dramatic decrease in muscle tension.

The kind of scene you choose depends on what has the most appeal to you. Some people choose the beach, a flower-filled meadow, a mountain stream, or an overlook with a great view. Pick a scene that appeals to you or one that you associate with peace, quiet, and renewal. Once you have decided on a place, close your eyes and try to fully imagine yourself being there, utilizing all of your senses. What do you hear? What do you see? What are you feeling? Imagine yourself fully enjoying the beauty of your surroundings and the experience of peace and quiet. Feel the warmth of the sun, breathe in the cool, fresh air, and listen to the wind in the trees. As an example, I'll describe a beach scene, which tends to be the scene chosen most frequently by the people I treat in my office.

> *Close your eyes. Imagine yourself on a quiet, deserted beach. No one else is allowed on your beach, so you're alone and safe. You are lying on the world's most comfortable beach chair. The weather is spectacular. The sky is blue, with just a few high, white, wispy clouds. The water is sparklingly clean, and you are enjoying watching and listening to the rhythm of the waves as they slowly roll up to the shore. It is so quiet. All you hear is the gentle pounding of the surf and the cries of a couple of*

seagulls. When you breathe in, you can taste the clean, slightly salty sea air. The air temperature is just right, and your body feels soothed by the sun and a light, cool breeze.

This is your beach. You don't have a care or worry in the world. This is your place to get away from it all, to soothe your soul and replenish your resources. If you find that other thoughts are intruding, actively visualize yourself pushing them away. Attach them to a cloud that is blowing offshore, or send them out with the outgoing tide. Keep your mind as empty as possible, just focusing on the peacefulness and comfort of the scene around you.

Whatever scene you choose, remember the elements of peacefulness, being far away from troubles and stressors, focusing on your physical senses, and fully experiencing your scene. Feel the warmth of the sun. Taste the clean, fresh air. Listen to the quiet, the trees whispering in the breeze, the birds chirping. Enjoy the beauty of the surroundings. Emphasize the safety and serenity of the scene.

Some people find it very difficult to empty their mind of disquieting thoughts. Some brains just seem to go at top speed all the time, and it takes a lot of effort to slow things down. If this is the case for you, take active steps to visualize your worrisome thoughts being banned or removed from your scene. Watch them moving downstream or being blown away by a strong wind. Tell yourself that you will deal with those things later, that this is your time for rest and to regain your resources. With practice and active effort, you will see significant improvement in your ability to clear your mind.

This type of relaxing visualization can be especially helpful to people who have been abused. Following a flashback of a traumatic memory, they may find it enormously soothing to visualize themselves in their "safe spot" to help to reduce the awful feeling of terror. For an abuse survivor, special emphasis should be placed on the fact that they are completely free from harm while in this safe place.

As a person with IBS, when you are utilizing calming visualization as a relaxation strategy, you may want to add another element: visualizing a body that is feeling healthy and free from physical discomfort. Your IBS and all that goes along with it are down at the bottom of the mountain, or well inland away from the beach. While in your quiet spot, you can imagine having a body that is comfortable, quiet, and relaxed.

Exercise: Deep Breathing

As part of an effort toward relaxing, it is often quite helpful to slow your breathing down into a nice, deep, regular rhythm. It is believed that an anxiety reaction is sometimes fueled by a bit of hyperventilation that occurs when a person is breathing in a rapid, shallow manner. Overbreathing results in an imbalance of the oxygen/carbon dioxide mix in your blood and can make you feel dizzy, faint, and light-headed, sweaty, tingly, or numb. It can also speed up your heart rate. All of these symptoms are typical of an anxiety attack. Slowing your breathing helps to ensure a healthy blood gas balance and works toward turning off that internal security alarm system.

As you are imagining yourself in your peaceful spot, focus on slowing down and regulating your breathing. Inhale slowly, through your nose, to a count of four. Exhale slowly through your mouth, also to the count of four. "In, two, three, four, and out two, three, four." An additional little anxiety-reducing trick is to say the word "relax" to yourself as you exhale. The word "relax" then becomes associated with a state of complete muscle relaxation and can be used as a cue to bring on the relaxed feeling quickly. So say to yourself, "In, two, three, four," and "Relax, two, three, four." Take a moment to practice this for a count of five breaths, in and out.

Now that you have got the counting part under your belt, you will need to learn to breathe deeply using your abdomen and diaphragm. Many people are chest breathers, which contributes to overbreathing and those uncomfortable physical symptoms of anxiety. When practicing your deep breathing, make sure you are wearing loose, comfortable clothes. Place one hand on your chest and the other on your abdomen, with your pinky finger just above your belly button. Think of your diaphragm as a balloon that will be filled with and emptied of air. As you inhale, focus on filling your diaphragm, and it will push your lower hand out. When you exhale, focus on emptying and relaxing your diaphragm. Throughout your inhales and exhales, your upper hand should remain fairly still. If you are a habitual chest breather, it may take some practice to keep those chest muscles relaxed and to use your abdomen to do the work. Try combining your counting and diaphragmatic breathing for a series of five breaths.

Incorporate your breathing into your visualization of your peaceful place. You can time your breathing to the comings and goings of the waves or the puffs of wind through the trees. As you exhale, you can visualize the tension draining from your body and going out to sea, off with an errant leaf, or down the river. As the tension drifts away, you are left with a peaceful, relaxed, comfortable body.

Exercise: Progressive Muscle Relaxation

Way back in 1929, a man named Jacobsen first developed a series of exercises that actively works to relax all of the muscle groups in the body. These exercises are simple to do and enable you to consciously reduce the amount of physical tension in your body.

To see how this works, take a moment to clench your fist. Count to three and then relax the muscles in your hand. Focus on the difference in the sensation of tension versus relaxation. It is this nice feeling of relaxation that we want you to feel all over your body.

Although there are many ways to do progressive muscle relaxation exercises, I prefer to have my patients start with the muscle groups at the top of their body and work their way down. This method helps a person to feel the tension drain from the body, replaced by a spreading feeling of warmth and relaxation. You may want to make a tape of the following instructions to listen to as you go through the exercises. Wear loose clothing, find a comfortable chair, and let yourself go.

> *To start, make a frown, tightening the muscles in your forehead. Hold for three seconds, then relax. Smooth out the tension, leaving your forehead feeling unwrinkled and relaxed. Screw up your eyes for three seconds, one, two, three, and then relax, leaving your eyelids feeling very heavy. Crinkle your nose for three seconds, then relax. Clench your jaw, one, two, three, and relax. Focus on keeping all of the muscles in your face relaxed. Feel the tension draining downward, leaving all of the muscles feeling warm, heavy and relaxed. Imagine that the warm sun is massaging away all of your tension and worries.*
>
> *Feel the sensation of relaxation moving slowly throughout your body. If the muscles in your neck feel tense, slowly turn your head to one side, gently stretching your neck muscles. Gently turn your head back to the front and slowly turn to the other side. Straighten your head one more time and imagine your neck muscles feeling loose and relaxed.*
>
> *Shrug your shoulders, hold them up toward your ears for the count of three, and then relax them. Make fists and tighten all of the muscles in your arms, and then relax them so that your arms are hanging limply by your side. Feel the tension draining from your shoulders, down your arms, and filling your arms and your hands with the sensation of warmth and relaxation.*

Take a deep breath in, tightening the muscles of your abdomen. As you exhale, let go of all of the tension in your upper body. You are now lying there feeling as loose and relaxed as a rag doll.

Tighten the muscles in your legs, pointing your toes toward the ceiling. Hold for three seconds and then relax. Feel the tension draining from your upper body, down your legs, and out through your toes. Your legs are now lying limp and loose; they feel warm, heavy, and relaxed.

As you sit there, does any part of your body still feel tense? Go back to that muscle group, tense it up, and then relax it. Focus on the pleasurable feeling that is associated with a relaxed muscle. Visualize the muscle tension draining from that area, leaving behind a feeling of warmth and heaviness. Imagine the sun massaging away the tension from those muscles.

Spend a few minutes enjoying the serenity of having a peaceful, relaxed body. Keep your breathing steady, exhaling away all unwanted tension. Fully experience your quiet scene, replenishing your spirit with its beauty. Relax.

When you are first learning the exercises, I recommend that you tense each muscle group in turn and then focus on relaxing it. Once you have mastered the skill, you can skip the step of tensing your muscle first, and just focus on progressively relaxing each muscle group, working your way down your body.

Keep an Eye on Anxiety

As you go through your day, try to have an awareness of how anxious or tense you feel. Practice your relaxation exercises twice a day, and you will see a reduction in your overall baseline anxiety level. If you find yourself feeling tense or stressed out, take the time to take a few deep breaths, relax your muscles, and reduce your anxiety level. Like that boxer we were talking about, you will find yourself to be a more mellow person, better equipped to handle whatever life throws at you.

On your self-monitoring sheets, you have been recording the severity of your IBS symptoms. You may find it helpful to record the severity of your anxiety as well, using a scale of 1 to 10. Doing this will help you to monitor your progress in anxiety management. Many of my patients will come in for their session with an anxiety level of 9 or 10. Without the use of any magic beans, a run-through of relaxation exercises usually results in an anxiety level of 1 or 2. That is a heck of a lot more comfortable!

Matthew is a thirty-five-year-old advertising executive who swears by relaxation exercises. Because his job is very high pressure and fast paced, his struggle with the symptoms of IBS was having a significant impact on his job performance. Matthew had always been an avid athlete, but the time requirements of his job were preventing him from spending much time working off his stress through physical exercise. For this reason the physical nature of relaxation exercises really appealed to him. Before and after work he took the time to fully relax himself. Throughout his work day, he monitored himself for signs of tension and then immediately kicked in some relaxation strategy. He found that taking deep breaths and relaxing all of his muscles on the exhale worked very well for him. He also found that by keeping his body as relaxed as possible, his IBS quieted down significantly. He is grateful to have learned a technique that not only keeps his IBS manageable but has been so helpful to him in coping with the demands of his job.

Learn to Assert Yourself

Assertiveness, in a nutshell, means standing up for yourself. It involves recognizing your feelings, rights, and preferences and expressing these to other people. There is some evidence that many people who suffer from IBS have difficulty expressing their anger. When something bothers them, they keep it all stuffed inside, and it is possible that this has a negative effect on their intestinal system. If you fall into this category, you will find it quite helpful to learn skills to better express your emotions.

I once read an interview with a woman who had recently retired from the world of professional women's basketball. She stated that her time on the court had prepared her well for the business world, due to the fact that in the world of sports, roles and rules are well defined; a goalie has the job of protecting the goal, a shortstop has a certain area of the field to cover, a quarterback calls and initiates each football play. There is usually an assigned space that each athlete functions in, and each sport has its own universally accepted set of rules. In life, each of us have various roles that we play. We each maintain a certain amount of personal space. In addition to the written rules of life, such as the law and Emily Post's etiquette, there is also a generally agreed-upon but unspoken set of rules for appropriate behavior. When we feel that another person is overstepping the bounds, violating one of these rules, or invading our personal space, we react with some negative emotion. Assertiveness is one way to handle that negative emotion, by expressing our displeasure to the other person. In a basketball game, the referee would cry, "Foul!"

Who Needs It, and When?

Assertiveness training is good for two different kinds of people. The obvious ones are people who are too passive in their approach to the world. They have difficulty speaking up to others, keep their feelings to themselves, and often view themselves as weak. Assertiveness training is also recommended for people with chronic anger control difficulties. These are people who deal with every situation with an aggressive approach. Assertiveness training helps these individuals learn to deal with a situation in a more moderate way so that conflict is more likely to be defused rather than escalated.

Many people don't like confrontation, so they shy away from it. The problem with this approach is that it may leave a person with unresolved feelings of anger and resentment that are just not good for physical and mental health. Assertiveness helps because it offers an outlet for these feelings. It also maximizes your chances of working out an acceptable solution with the other person because it's designed to reduce defensiveness on their part.

The only problem is that assertiveness doesn't always work. Some people are defensive, hostile, or aggressive, no matter how you approach them. They don't react to you poorly because you aren't tough enough, but because that's how they treat everyone. What you want to do is learn the skills necessary to consider yourself an assertive person. Then you can make the decision as to what is in your best interest. Is it in your best interest to speak up? Will it alert the other person to your feelings so that they'll act in a more considerate manner next time? Does it feel good just to say "ouch," even if it really won't change anything? Is it not even worth the trouble to say anything? Is it safer not to confront the other person because of a good chance of physical violence? The point is that you are making the decision based on what is ultimately in your best interest, rather than keeping quiet due to a lack of skills or confidence.

When to be assertive? Look to your self-monitoring sheets for feedback. Look under your Feelings column. Are you feeling angry, resentful, or overwhelmed? Would speaking up help you feel better? Remember that our emotional responses give us information regarding how we are reacting to the goings-on around us. Listen to your inner voice and solve problems accordingly. In order to successfully assert yourself, you need to have a thorough awareness of your internal thoughts and feelings. You've been working on this ever since chapter 6. Listen to your internal reactions to the world and figure out what your needs, desires, and preferences are, then base your assertiveness on this information.

Start with "I"

In order to maximize success and minimize defensiveness, you want to begin your assertion with an expression of your own feelings. Use statements that begin with the word "I" and follow the "I" with an expression of your feelings or preferences. "I felt angry today when you didn't even ask how it went at the doctor's," or "I would prefer that in the future you take a more active interest in my treatment." When you use an "I" statement, you give the other person an implied out, or a way to save face. You are not specifically telling them that they did anything wrong, you are just telling them how you felt or reacted to what they did or didn't do. On the other hand, when you start a confrontation with the word "You," you almost automatically put the other person in a position to have to defend themselves. You can easily see that a statement such as "I was angry when you joked about my IBS in front of all of your friends" is bound to have a very different outcome than "You are such a boor!" The basic recipe for assertiveness comes down to a simple A, B, C: I feel A, when you do B, and I would prefer that in the future you do C.

Accentuate the Positive

There are other useful techniques to keep in mind. It often helps to start your assertion with a focus on something positive. This reduces defensiveness and sets the tone for easier conflict resolution. Express your desires in the form of preferences, as opposed to demands. Rather than telling the other person what to do, you are simply requesting that they think about honoring your wishes. Work to see the other person's point of view. The four magic words for bringing a fight to a close are "I can see that." Once the other person feels that their point of view has been acknowledged, they will generally be much more open to hearing your side of things. Try to come up with a compromise that lets everyone feel okay about the way things have been worked out.

Keep in mind that most people don't do what they do just to tick you off. Most perceived transgressions occur just because of how people walk through this world. People with different personalities and different agendas are bound to clash. When someone inadvertently steps on your toes, say "ouch" and ask them not to do it again. If it is the nature of their personality to keep doing so, then you need to come to grips with this and figure out different ways of coping rather than continuing to complain each time they keep on doing the same boneheaded thing.

Setting Limits

In addition to being a way to resolve conflict, assertiveness also has to do with setting limits on the behavior of others. It means maintaining your position in line, asking someone to stop talking during a movie, or asking to speak with a manager. Assertiveness means asking a doctor to explain things until you understand. It means sticking up for your rights. You have every right to do so and all it takes is some practice. Start small. Many people find it easier to be assertive with strangers as opposed to family and friends, as they feel they have less to lose. Practice on the hostess of your favorite restaurant and *then* take on your mother-in-law. Each time you successfully stand up for yourself, pat yourself on the back. Like other behaviors, an assertive response is more likely to be repeated if it is met with a reward.

Holding Your Own

Being assertive doesn't mean that you have to develop an aggressive personality. Similarly, you can be an assertive person even if you are in the shadow of a domineering personality. I worked with a lovely woman named Delores who suffers from IBS. She described herself as a "meek, weak person." When I asked her what she based this on, she stated that she had difficulty standing up to her husband and let him take control when they were out in public. She described her husband as being loud, overbearing, and confrontational. She stated that he frequently made a scene when out in stores or restaurants, while she stood quietly by. When I asked her questions about how she handled things when he wasn't around, for example when she was at work, or when she felt that she wasn't getting proper service at a store, she replied that she generally was able to speak up. I told her that it seemed to me that she was an assertive person but that she confused being loud and confrontational with being strong. As trees show us, strength lies in flexibility, and Delores struck me as very flexible. Her strategy of standing by quietly while her husband ranted and raved was actually a very smart one. If he chose to let himself get all worked up and carried away, that was his problem. She didn't need to get involved.

With this perspective in mind, Delores has found these outbursts of her husband to be much less stressful. Instead of standing next to him feeling foolish, and beating up on herself for remaining silent, she now stays calm and waits for the storm to pass. While using this strategy, she has been pleased to note that her intestines are not set off quite so frequently. She is no longer filled with self-doubt and is learning to better cope with her husband's personality without letting it take such a toll on her.

Practice Gradual Exposure

When a person experiences a traumatic event, they become sensitized or overreactive to stimuli that were associated with the trauma. A war veteran might experience fear and panic in response to a sudden loud noise. A person who was in a car accident that occurred when it was raining might experience heightened anxiety when driving on wet pavement. A person with IBS might associate certain places or situations with abdominal pain and distress, and suffer from debilitating anticipatory anxiety.

Avoidance Isn't the Answer

In response to the heightened anxiety brought on by stimuli that were present at the time of the trauma, many people choose avoidance as a coping strategy. Avoidance is rewarded by the absence of anxiety. The downside to avoidance is not only that it restricts one's life but that it enables the association between the feared stimuli and the resulting anxiety to remain strong. Gradual exposure is the direct antidote for avoidance because it involves slowly facing up to your fears.

For some IBS sufferers, avoidance becomes so all-encompassing that life becomes narrow, restricted, and lonely. Your self-monitoring sheets should give you some feedback as to the type of situations you might be avoiding. Slowly reintroducing yourself to these avoided places and situations can help you to break the association between them and the experience of pain and suffering. This will free you up to resume living a fulfilling, interesting life.

Taking It Step by Step

To illustrate the use of gradual exposure, let's take the example of a person who has experienced the trauma of being mauled by a dog. A gradual exposure approach might start with merely showing the individual pictures of a variety of dogs. The next step might be to have them view a dog from a bit of a distance. The person might then be ready to have limited contact with a puppy before eventually getting close to a larger dog.

Exposure helps people to overcome their fears. For example, the dog bite victim learns that not all dogs bite. Each time the fearful driver drives in the rain without an accident, their anxiety reaction is lessened. The veteran learns that loud noises are not necessarily life threatening. Claudia's story is an excellent example of the process of trauma, avoidance, exposure, and recovery.

Claudia was a twenty-eight-year-old who had worked as an executive secretary for a defense firm located in a suburban area. She came to see me because she felt that IBS had become a major obstacle in her life. Claudia told me that she had recently found the courage to leave the company where she had been working since high school in order to seek employment in the city, where she felt she would have the opportunity to earn more money. She sent out some résumés and was quickly called to interview with a brokerage in the financial district. To get to the interview, she had to take a train and then two buses, and she began to experience abdominal cramps while on the train. The cramps worsened as she traveled by bus. The urge to get to a bathroom became so urgent and intense that when she got to the building, she ran straight into the bathroom and experienced wave after wave of diarrhea. She felt so ill that she never made it to the appointment and eventually called a friend to come into the city and drive her home.

The trauma of this experience left Claudia with two major avoidance issues. She refused to take public transportation of any kind, and she became quite fearful of any type of scheduled appointment. She not only quit her job search, but even refused to schedule doctor appointments and dates with friends. Obviously her fears had a serious negative impact on her quality of life.

In order to help Claudia get her old life back, we set up two plans, known as hierarchies, to gradually expose her to the things she feared. They looked like this:

Hierarchy One—Public Transportation

1. Standing at bus stop for five minutes

2. Riding bus for one stop

3. Riding bus for two and eventually up to five stops

4. Riding train one stop
5. Riding train two to five stops
6. Taking express bus into the city
7. Taking train into the city

Hierarchy Two—Scheduled Appointments

1. Agree to meet friend for cup of coffee at designated time.
2. Make and keep appointment to get nails done.
3. Make and keep appointment to get a haircut.
4. Make and keep a dentist appointment.
5. Set up and attend a local job interview.
6. Set up and attend a job interview in the city.

By breaking down her goals into very small steps, Claudia was able to slowly work her way back into a normal life. We knew that her therapy was complete when she landed a great job with an accounting firm in the city at almost double her old salary!

Setting Personal Goals

Take a look at your self-monitoring sheets. Do you see a pattern in terms of the situations that you've been avoiding? Set some goals for yourself as to where you'd like to be operating more freely. Use your creativity to devise a hierarchy that gradually exposes you to the elements of your fears. Step by step, slowly face up to your demons.

Reward Yourself

Each time you successfully complete one of the tasks on your list, proudly cross it off and reward yourself. A reward can be a simple pat on the back, or, if your wallet allows, treat yourself to something indulgent. It doesn't matter what you choose—just make sure to acknowledge your accomplishment in some way.

Baby Steps

If you find yourself stuck on a particular step, see if it can be broken down even further into smaller steps. Claudia had difficulty taking the leap toward going on a job interview. As an interim step, she set the goal of attending an interview with a job placement service. This seemed less stressful to her because she wasn't interviewing for a specific job. After handling that situation without difficulty, she was able to move on to the next step and attend a real job interview. If you take a step and are unsuccessful, back up and repeat the last successful step. Then see if you can come up with a more achievable next step.

Visualization

You might find it helpful to use positive visualization prior to your actual attempts at exposure. After running through your relaxation exercises, take a moment to visualize yourself calmly performing the next item on your hierarchy. Walk yourself through the assigned task, step by step, in your imagination. See yourself successfully using your anxiety management skills to keep yourself and your body calm. You can use cognitive challenging, calming self-statements, deep breathing, and progressive muscle relaxation. This mental practice will help you maximize your chances for success when you face your fears in actuality. Use these same anxiety management skills when you're out there trying out hierarchy items. Aren't you impressed by how much you've learned?

Specialized Strategies

In addition to relaxation, assertiveness, and gradual exposure, two other behavioral strategies have been shown to be effective in reducing IBS symptoms, namely hypnosis and biofeedback. Neither of them is anywhere near as intimidating as they sound, but you do need a trained professional to administer the therapy. Before choosing a therapist, make sure that they have experience and knowledge regarding the treatment of IBS. Here is a short overview of what is involved with these two specialized treatments.

Hypnosis

Hypnosis in real life is not so far removed from the way it's portrayed in cartoons. The therapist uses one of a variety of hypnotic techniques to induce a trance state (an altered state of consciousness) in the subject. Generally this occurs due to an extremely deep state of relaxation. While the subject is in the hypnotic state, the hypnotist makes therapeutic suggestions. These suggestions may consist of changes in behavior, sensation, or thoughts. Hypnosis has been used successfully for smoking cessation, for improved control over eating, and for dealing with many medical conditions. For a person with health problems, such as IBS, suggestions made to the subject while in the trance state would include strategies for dealing with pain and coping with symptoms.

Biofeedback

Biofeedback is actually kind of fun. The purpose of biofeedback is to give you feedback regarding bodily processes that you aren't usually aware of. In order to get this feedback, you get hooked up to electronic devices that measure things such as heart rate, skin temperature, blood pressure, and muscle tension. This is a painless, noninvasive procedure in which sensors are applied to the relevant parts of the body. A computer monitor then gives visual or auditory feedback regarding these measurements. It's a little like playing a video game, as you try to change the way your body is responding. The process helps you develop voluntary control over unhealthy or abnormal bodily processes. Biofeedback has been used successfully in treating a variety of disorders, such as headaches, attention deficit disorder, and asthma, and it's been shown to be effective in improved bowel control in patients with IBS.

Cataloging Your Coping Skills

You are now equipped with an extensive arsenal of skills to use for coping with and perhaps preventing those nasty IBS symptoms. In addition to the cognitive strategies you learned in the last chapter, you can now use and practice the skills of relaxation, assertiveness, and exposure to your fears. If you choose to go for the specialized treatments of hypnosis and biofeedback, you will have additional tools for coping with IBS. With all of your newfound knowledge, IBS shouldn't seem like such a scary beast. You no longer need to be ruled by your intestines, you no longer need to feel overwhelmed and intimidated by your body, and you can experience the proud feeling that comes with successful mastery of new skills. Continue to fill out your self-monitoring sheets as needed, with particular emphasis on your entries into that column on the right, as you catalogue your newfound coping skills!

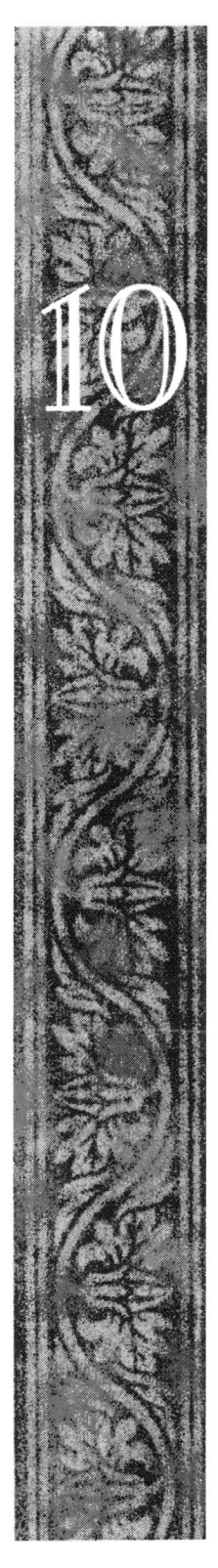

10 Beyond IBS: Developing a Healthy Lifestyle

A person's life should never be defined by just one thing. Unfortunately, when a physical ailment like IBS manifests itself, it sometimes becomes all encompassing. Everything revolves around the illness. Plans, work, family, and fun are all put on the back burner. The cruel irony is that this centralized attention actually serves to exacerbate the ills of IBS. The more attention you pay to the symptoms, worrying when they'll strike next, being hypervigilant about the presence of uncomfortable physical feelings, the worse you're likely to feel. Chronic worry and scanning for symptoms increase physiological arousal. This increased physiological arousal contributes to intestinal distress.

It's time to put IBS back in its place. You've learned strategies for coping with specific symptoms, handling difficult situations, and changing unhealthy ways of thinking and behaving. As an extension to all that you have learned, you can apply your skills toward an overall improvement in your quality of life, working toward a life that is full, rich, and satisfying.

Coping with a Chronic Illness

IBS is an illness with a chronic course. Like other chronic illnesses, it is comprised of episodes of exacerbation and periods of remission. Living a fulfilling life under these circumstances can be quite a challenge, but it's far from impossible. Patience, creativity, and a sense of humor can be your guides.

Whatever the illness or disability, anyone coping with a chronic condition will experience emotions similar to those of the grieving process. Certainly the loss of your health and trust in your body is worth grieving. As with reacting to a death, a person will experience times of sadness, anger, questioning, and challenges of faith. Take the time to mourn; you *do* have something to cry about. It's okay to get angry; it *is* unfair that this has happened to you. Feel what you need to feel and then shift your focus toward improved coping and carving out some good times for yourself.

Self-care is critical when you are coping with a chronic physical ailment. When you feel sick, soothe yourself. Make yourself comfortable and remind yourself that you'll feel better soon. Work to keep your overall stressors low and your body calm. If you make self-care your number-one priority, you'll feel better and find that you end up with a lot more to offer others.

Acknowledge your illness to yourself. You aren't just imagining things. You *are* ill, so cut yourself some slack. Acknowledgment is different from acceptance. You don't have to like this, and you don't have to eagerly embrace this particular cross. However, it *is* your current reality and you need to keep it in mind as you set reasonable expectations for yourself.

Acknowledge your illness to others. Telling people about what you are experiencing will open the door to helpful support and educate others about what it's like to cope with a chronic condition. If you cancel an outing because you're ill, being honest will prevent others from thinking that you canceled because you don't like them! Don't be too proud to ask for help. Most people love to do things for others; it makes them feel good and helps free up access to *your* help when *they* need it. Opening up to others about your struggle can help to forge deeper bonds that are good for your body and your soul.

One of the biggest challenges of most chronic illnesses is that their episodic nature wreaks havoc on planning. Plan away anyway! Use all of your skills to help yourself successfully follow through on your plans. If you feel well, have a great time. If you aren't so lucky, give yourself credit for having tried, and remind yourself that you won't feel this way forever.

Don't view exacerbations as failures. The coping skills you've developed are designed to reduce the frequency, intensity, and duration of your symptoms, but they are not a cure. You are still going to get sick sometimes. Nurse yourself, but don't berate yourself for not coping well enough. Remember, you're having an ongoing battle with biology. Focus on the gains you've made, the skills you've learned that you never had before, and the places and people you were able to enjoy because of the better symptom control you've developed. Again, acknowledge the reality of your condition.

Stress Management

My patients always laugh when their doctors ask them, in response to elevated blood pressure, a relapse of IBS, or the occurrence of chronic headaches, if they have been under stress. They reply, "Of course!" and think to themselves, "Who isn't?" Yes, life in the modern world can be stressful. But dealing with the stressors in your life doesn't have to be a passive process. There are steps you can take to actively cope with, rather than feel overwhelmed by, the onslaught.

Relaxation

This is an area where you're already a pro. Using relaxation exercises on a regular basis keeps your system operating in a calm way. A healthier, relaxed body is much better equipped to deal with whatever life throws at it.

Learn to Prioritize

We all get overwhelmed when we have too much to do and not enough time to do it. If you're feeling swamped, you have two choices: prioritize or delegate. In order to prioritize, you need to take a moment to ask yourself which things are the most pressing or important. Instead of running around like a chicken without a head, take five minutes to make a list. It can be exhausting and overwhelming for your brain to try to hold on to all the important bits of information regarding what has to be done. Writing it down can bring some relief, as you no longer have to work to try not to forget anything. Place the most important items, or the ones with more immediate deadlines, at the top of the list. Anything that is not quite so important, or that can wait, should be placed on the bottom. Look at the first few items on the list, think about your schedule, and figure out how things can be best fit in. Each time you complete a task, cross it off so that you feel the rewarding pleasure that comes with accomplishment. This will also make your list shorter, which will help you to feel calmer.

Downsizing May Be the Answer

If you are overwhelmed with stressors, remember the word "downsize." Companies downsize when they feel their expenses are too high and they need to be run more efficiently. You can successfully downsize by letting unimportant things go. Maybe your closets don't have to be so organized, maybe you don't have to vacuum every day, maybe you can throw out those items at the bottom of your In box that you haven't gotten to in the last six months. In the overall scheme of things, how bad is it to just let some things go? If it means that you will feel healthier, then allow yourself to use short-cuts: only clean the rooms that you use, order take-out food. Let go of unrealistic standards and free yourself up to spend more of your time doing the things that you like to do, instead of always feeling bogged down by the things that you think you ought to do.

It's Okay to Delegate

When people are stressed out, it's usually not because of a lack of competence in handling life but simply because they have too much to do. The strongest weight lifters in the world reach a point at which they cannot lift an additional ounce. The inability to lift that heavy weight in no way means that they are weak. Similarly, a person's inability to handle everything on their plate does not imply weakness, just a need to seek assistance.

Ask for help! Don't fall into the trap that if you don't do it yourself it will never get done or it won't get done right. Sometimes good enough is good enough. Think of the time saved as the trade-off for less than perfect results. Be a smart delegator. Assess who has the skills or the personality to get the job done, then match the task with the person who is most likely to be able to do a good job with it.

Don't concern yourself with being a burden to others. As noted previously, most people love to help. It makes them feel good and frees them up to ask for your help when they need it. All you need to do is make a polite request. Be reasonable, and people will most likely respond positively. Remember that they have the right to say "no." If they agree to your request, express your gratitude and then don't second-guess yourself. If they say "yes," it means that they have willingly decided that this is something that is manageable for them. If they didn't want to do it, or thought it was too much, they would have declined. If someone does decline, accept it gratefully and adjust your expectations accordingly for the future.

Responsibility and Control

We touched on this concept earlier in the book. Many people feel responsible for everything! It is not hard to see why these folks end up feeling overwhelmed. Just remember: If you don't have control over something, you aren't responsible for it. A great illustration of this is to think about the effort that it takes to plan a wedding. Most people find this process to be very stressful; in fact, marrying off a daughter ranks pretty high on those lists of stressful life events. Planning a wedding is overwhelming in part because there are so many details to attend to. The planners feel responsible for everything. However, there are countless stories of weddings that have gone awry: catering halls that go out of business two weeks before, brides who faint during the ceremony, cakes that don't get delivered. None of these events are the fault of the planners, as it is impossible for anyone to have total control over an outcome. All the planners can do is make reasonably good arrangements and then simply hope for the best.

This way of thinking about the relationship between control and responsibility is applicable to all kinds of human situations. One of the main things that we don't have control over is the behavior of other people. So if someone else chooses to behave in an inappropriate way, remember that it's not a reflection on you. This kind of detachment will make you a lot calmer if you find yourself related, either by birthright or choice, to someone who behaves in a manner that doesn't always make you feel comfortable.

Just Say No

The most obvious way to prevent being overwhelmed by your responsibilities is to not take them on in the first place. Be kind to yourself and decline requests that you know have the potential to be the straw that breaks your back. It can be a challenge to strike a balance between the desire to be a helpful friend, citizen, and employee and your need to be healthy. If you take on too much and you suffer for it, either physically or emotionally, it's not good for anyone. Don't feel that if you don't do something, terrible consequences will ensue. One way or another, things get done and everyone survives. Don't let your health be the price you pay for the belief that you are so important. You *are* important, just because you're you, not because you're essential for the well-being of the rest of the world.

When balancing your obligations to others, it is helpful to think of the balance in terms of wants and needs. If you are responsible for other individuals, whether they are children, elderly parents, or sick relatives, remember that you are only obligated to make sure that their needs are met. Remember this: Their needs should come before your wants, but your needs should come before their wants. You have a need for sleep, rest, and pleasurable activities. You are under no obligation to sacrifice all of these things to satisfy every one of their desires. You decide which of their demands represent needs as opposed to wants. This perspective will greatly relieve you of unnecessary guilt and help you to feel more comfortable with the decisions that you make.

Increasing Physical Activity

Participation in physical fitness is once again on the rise. If you're already exercising on a regular basis, good for you! If not, here's the best reason yet to start: exercise releases endorphins, those happy, pain-relieving chemicals in our brains. Endorphins relax the muscles in the intestinal system. Relax the muscles, reduce spasms, and regulate transit time, and you may find that your bowel is not quite so irritable.

Start Moving

To get yourself started, don't focus too much on the word exercise. It often conjures up ugly images of huffing and puffing or the trauma of gym class. Focus instead on increasing your level of physical activity. Use your body more, so that it feels better. Do what you like to do. Do you like to garden, walk around and see what your neighbors are doing to their houses, or work your body up into a good sweat? Whatever it is that you like, do more and more of it.

Vary your routine. Listen to your inner voice and set reasonable goals for increasing the duration or intensity of whatever activity you choose. Exercise experts recommend a program where you focus more on cardiovascular exercises one day and then strength training, using weights to strengthen and tone muscles, the next. Besides being good for your body, this varied routine helps keep you from being bored or seeing exercise as a chore.

The Pleasure Principle

Be social. Nothing is more motivating than sharing your progress or interest with a friend. And there is no easier way to make friends, or meet that certain someone, than by sharing an interest in the same activity. Meet a friend to go out walking, join a gym and take some classes, or hook up with a local running or bicycling club. You will meet people who are enjoying life, become a part of that, and share the wealth.

Stick with it. Those great endorphins get released approximately twenty minutes after you begin to engage in vigorous exercise. This means that if you stick with the early huffing and puffing, you may actually feel better the longer you keep going. Again, start small, but add on as you feel comfortable, with the goal of enjoying that endorphin rush. You'll find that the good feeling you get from exercising is fairly long lasting, partially due to biology and partially due to a proud feeling of accomplishment and self-care.

Don't Give Up

The other reason to stick with it is that it may take three to six months after starting an exercise regimen before you begin to see real changes in your body. Again, the more immediate results are better self-esteem, pride in accomplishment, and learning to enjoy what your body has to offer. If you stick it out for three to six months, you'll see muscle definition that will make you vain, a body that handles routine tasks with ease (you know, something as simple as getting out of a chair), and significant progress as to the length and difficulty of your workouts.

Schedule time for exercise into your daily routine. Make it a priority, like finding time to brush your teeth or getting to work on time. Pick a time that is reasonable and that works for you. Some people love to exercise in the morning, because it gives them a charge that lasts throughout the day. If this works for you, you'll find yourself loving the fact that you had your own time, before giving your time away to others as you go through your day. On the other hand, if you are barely able to drag yourself out of bed in the morning, then it's foolish to think that you'll get up forty-five minutes earlier to exercise. Many people swear by exercise at the end of the day to work off the day's stress and tension. Exercise is a wonderful way to shift gears from the demands of the day into the leisure of the evening. When it's time for bed, your body is pleasantly fatigued and proudly relaxed.

Increase the overall time you use your body. Climb the stairs instead of using the elevator, and take a parking space that's a few feet away rather than waiting for someone in a close space to pull out. Go for a walk on your lunch hour. Go out dancing instead of going to a movie. Play volleyball on the beach. Use your body to have fun. It's a heck of a lot better than viewing your body as the enemy.

Your Body, Your Friend

Speaking of viewing your body as the enemy, if you're one of those people who struggles constantly with your weight, exercise is a wonderful way to become reacquainted with your body as a friend. Shift your focus away from weight loss and focus instead on helping your body to work smoothly and feel better. Prevailing research suggests that body type and body size are strongly influenced by genetics. We unfortunately live in a society where the ideal body shape is at direct odds with a body that is healthy for most people. Stop feeling like a failure for not living up to these unrealistic societal expectations and work with your body to strengthen it so that it works better for you. It goes back to that acknowledge/accept concept again. You don't have to like the fact that your body isn't shaped the way that you would prefer. Acknowledge that a thin body might not be realistic for you and set your sights on regular, healthy use of your body so that you can feel good about yourself.

Just for Fun

All work and no play isn't good for anyone. Coping with a highly reactive digestive system can be hard work. You'll feel a lot better if you offset all that work with some activities and experiences that are designed to bring you some pure pleasure.

In an adult life, responsibilities can be numerous, and as we've been discussing, at times they can be overwhelming or all encompassing. People often lose sight of what brings them joy, happiness, or a feeling of well-being. They forget what it means to have fun or what it feels like to have a good belly laugh. Excuses are easy to find, as in "I just don't have the time," but just as time is carved out for obligations, time can be carved out for pleasure, if it is made a priority.

To get in touch with what you like doing, think back to your childhood. What are your happiest memories? What were you doing? When you hear other people relating stories about their experiences, what appeals to you? What makes you feel envious? Again, listen to your inner voice or gut reaction and get in touch with your preferences and desires. Read through the following list and check off any items that appeal to your sense of play, pleasure, or adventure:

- Walk through a park.
- Sit on a beach.
- Take a long, hot bath.
- Call a friend.
- Go out for ice cream.
- Hold a baby.
- Sail a boat.
- Rent a funny movie.
- Climb a mountain.
- Write a letter to an old friend.

- Call your mother.
- Take a train ride.
- Sit in a hot tub.
- Ride a bike.
- Fly a kite.
- Curl up with a good book.
- Cook a gourmet meal.
- Paint a picture.
- Browse through a bookstore.
- Go fishing.
- Learn a foreign language.

The list could be endless. Reward yourself with the simple pleasures in life. If you have to do something that is difficult, painful, or heart wrenching, follow it up with something that is enjoyable. Work to enrich your life, filling it with fun, people, and challenges. Counteract the restrictions placed on you by your IBS. Break free and live a little!

From All Bad Things . . .

So, IBS has been a bummer. You didn't ask for it and you certainly didn't deserve it. Well, take a moment to congratulate yourself. Give yourself a big pat on the back for turning adversity into triumph. Your illness has served as the motivation for you to learn healthier ways of living. The benefits that you will enjoy from having made the changes that were necessitated by your IBS will be with you for a lifetime. What are these benefits?

Number one, you've made changes that have overall health benefits. You are eating more carefully—and foods that are much healthier—rather than the ones that your body can no longer tolerate. You are keeping your body relaxed and managing your stressors so that they no longer take such a toll on your body.

You should be enjoying the benefits of improved mental health as well. Stress management and relaxation techniques help to reduce the possibility of burnout and breakdowns. You have learned how to better listen to yourself, identifying and using your emotions in a helpful way, and classifying and meeting your desires so that you'll feel more satisfied with the way things go.

Having the best quality of life in any possible circumstances is what it's all about. Your assertiveness and comfort in talking openly about your IBS will help you to have easier, more enjoyable relationships with others. Treating your body well, through avoiding exposure to triggers and increasing your physical activity, will significantly improve your overall comfort level. It is said that the best revenge is a life well lived. Seek revenge against IBS, break free from its chains, and have a great life.

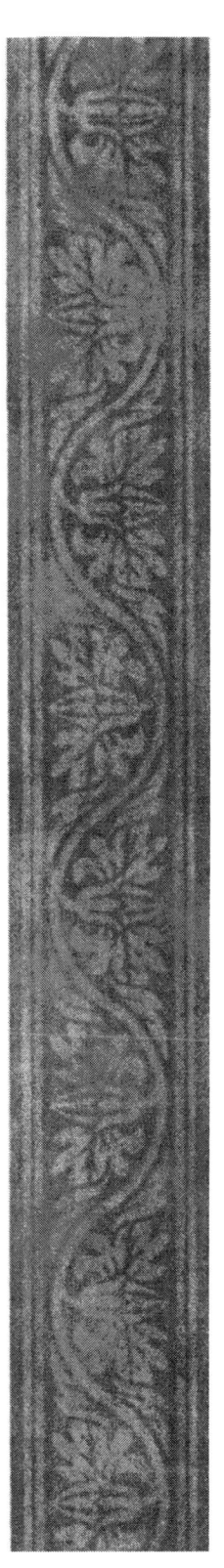

RESOURCES

International Foundation for Functional Gastrointestinal Disorders
P.O. Box 17864
Milwaukee, WI 53217
Toll-free number: 888-964-2001

National Digestive Diseases Information Clearinghouse
2 Information Way
Bethesda, MD 20892-3570
(301) 654-3810

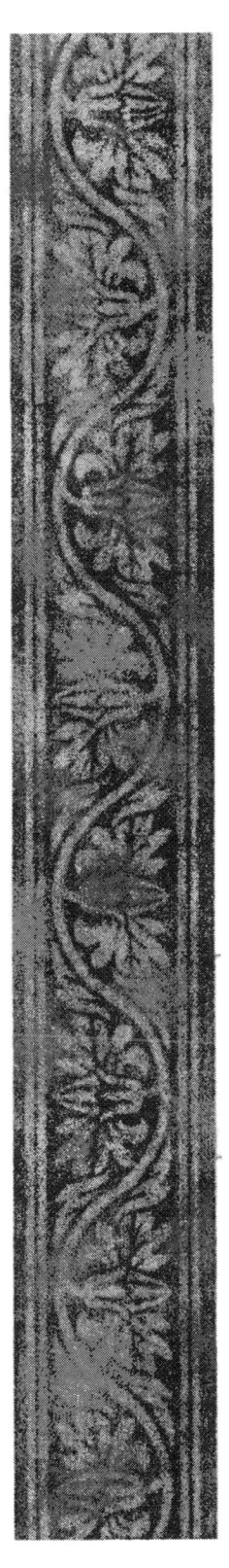

REFERENCES

Cook, I. J., A. Van Eeden, and S. M. Collins. 1987. Patients with irritable bowel syndrome have greater pain tolerance than normal subjects. *Gastroenterology* 93:727-733.

Craighead, L. W., and H. N. Allen. 1995. Appetite awareness training: A cognitive-behavioral intervention for binge eating. *Cognitive and Behavioral Practice* 2:249-270.

Creed, F., T. Craig, and R. Farmer. 1988. Functional abdominal pain, psychiatric illness, and life events. *Gut* 29:235-242.

DiPalma, J. A., M. S. Jackson, B. A. Tolliver, E. D. Barnett, and J. F. Allen. 1994. Does lactose maldigestion play a role in irritable bowel syndrome. *Gastroenterology* 106:A488.

Drossman, D. A., J. Leserman, G. Nachman, Z. Li, H. Gluck, T. C. Toomey, and C. M. Mitchell. 1990. Sexual and physical abuse in women with functional or organic gastrointestinal disorders. *Annals of Internal Medicine* 113:828-833.

Drossman, D. S., D. C. McKee, R. S. Sandler, C. M. Mitchell, E. M. Cramer, B. C. Lowman, and A. L. Burger. 1988. Psychosocial factors in the irritable bowel syndrome: A multivariate study of patients and nonpatients with irritable bowel syndrome. *Gastroenterology* 95:701-708.

Farthing, M. 1995. Irritable bowel, irritable body, or irritable brain? *British Medical Journal* 310:171-176.

Francis, C. Y., and P. J. Whorwell. 1994. Bran and irritable bowel syndrome: Time for reappraisal. *Lancet* 344:39-41.

Harvey, R. F., E. C. Mauad, and A. M. Brown. 1987. Prognosis in the irritable bowel syndrome: A 5-year prospective study. *Lancet* 1:963-965.

Jacobsen, E. 1929. *Progressive Relaxation*. Chicago: University of Chicago Press.

Jones, V. A., P. McLaughlin, M. Shorthouse, E. Workman, and J. O. Hunter. 1982. Food intolerance: A major factor in the pathogenesis of irritable bowel syndrome. *Lancet* ii:1116-1117.

Kellow, J. E., R. C. Gill, and D. L. Wingate. 1990. Prolonged ambulent recordings of small bowel motility demonstrating abnormalities in the irritable bowel syndrome. *Gastroenterology* 98:1208-1218.

Mayer, E. A., and G. F. Gebhart. 1994. Basic and clinical aspects of visceral hyperalgesia. *Gastroenterology* 107:271-293.

Neal, K. R., J. Hebden, and R. Spiller. 1997. Prevalence of gastrointestinal symptoms six months after bacterial gastroenteritis and risk factors for development of the irritable bowel syndrome: postal survey of patients. *British Medical Journal* 314:779-783.

Smith, R. C., D. S. Greenbaum, J. B. Vancouver, R. C. Henry, M. A. Reinhart, R. B. Greenbaum, H. A. Dean, and J. E. Mayle. 1990. Psychosocial factors are associated with health care seeking rather than diagnosis in irritable bowel syndrome. *Gastroenterology* 98:293-301.

Thompson, W. G. 1993. Irritable bowel syndrome: Pathogenesis and management. *Lancet* 341:1569-1572.

Whitehead, W. E., L. J. Cheskin, B. R. Heller, J. C. Robinson, M. D. Crowell, C. Benjamin, and M. M. Schuster. 1990. Evidence for exacerbation of irritable bowel syndrome during menses. *Gastroenterology* 98:1485-1489.

Whitehead, W. E., M. D. Crowell, J. C. Robinson, B. R. Heller, and M. M. Schuster. 1992. Effects of stressful life events on bowel symptoms: Subjects with irritable bowel syndrome compared with subjects without bowel dysfunction. *Gut* 33:825-830.

Some Other New Harbinger Titles

A Cancer Patient's Guide to Overcoming Depression and Anxiety, Item 5044 $19.95
The Diabetes Lifestyle Book, Item 5167 $16.95
Solid to the Core, Item 4305 $14.95
Staying Focused in the Age of Distraction, Item 433X $16.95
Living Beyond Your Pain, Item 4097 $19.95
Fibromyalgia & Chronic Fatigue Syndrome, Item 4593 $14.95
Your Miraculous Back, Item 4526 $18.95
TriEnergetics, Item 4453 $15.95
Emotional Fitness for Couples, Item 4399 $14.95
The MS Workbook, Item 3902 $19.95
Depression & Your Thyroid, Item 4062 $15.95
The Eating Wisely for Hormonal Balance Journal, Item 3945 $15.95
Healing Adult Acne, Item 4151 $15.95
The Memory Doctor, Item 3708 $11.95
The Emotional Wellness Way to Cardiac Health, Item 3740 $16.95
The Cyclothymia Workbook, Item 383X $18.95
The Matrix Repatterning Program for Pain Relief, Item 3910 $18.95
Transforming Stress, Item 397X $10.95
Eating Mindfully, Item 3503 $13.95
Living with RSDS, Item 3554 $16.95
The Ten Hidden Barriers to Weight Loss, Item 3244 $11.95
The Sjogren's Syndrome Survival Guide, Item 3562 $15.95
Stop Feeling Tired, Item 3139 $14.95
Responsible Drinking, Item 2949 $19.95
The Mitral Valve Prolapse/Dysautonomia Survival Guide, Item 3031 $14.95
The Vulvodynia Survival Guide, Item 2914 $16.95
The Multifidus Back Pain Solution, Item 2787 $12.95
Move Your Body, Tone Your Mood, Item 2752 $17.95
The Trigger Point Therapy Workbook, Item 2507 $19.95

Call **toll free, 1-800-748-6273,** or log on to our online bookstore at www.newharbinger.com to order. Have your Visa or Mastercard number ready. Or send a check for the titles you want to New Harbinger Publications, Inc., 5674 Shattuck Ave., Oakland, CA 94609. Include $4.50 for the first book and 75¢ for each additional book, to cover shipping and handling. (California residents please include appropriate sales tax.) Allow two to five weeks for delivery.

Prices subject to change without notice.

Made in the USA
Middletown, DE
03 March 2023

26128087R00102